Angina

FOURTH EDITION

Graham Jackson FRCP FESC FACC
Consultant Cardiologist
Guy's and St Thomas' Hospitals
London, UK

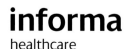

informa
healthcare

First edition published in the United Kingdom in 1991 by Martin Dunitz Ltd, 7–9 Pratt Street, London NW1 0AE. Second edition published in 1995. Third edition published in 2000.

Fourth edition published in the United Kingdom in 2008 by Informa Healthcare, Telephone House, 69–77 Paul Street, London EC2A 4LQ. Informa Healthcare is a trading division of Informa UK Ltd. Registered Office: 37/41 Mortimer Street, London W1T 3JH. Registered in England and Wales Number 1072954.

Tel.: +44 (0)20 7017 5000
Fax.: +44 (0)20 7017 6699
Website: www.informahealthcare.com

A CIP record for this book is available from the British Library.
Library of Congress Cataloging-in-Publication Data

Data available on application

ISBN 10: 1 84184 669 4
ISBN 13: 978 1 84184 669 9

Distributed in North and South America by
Taylor & Francis
6000 Broken Sound Parkway, NW (Suite 300)
Boca Raton, FL 33487, USA

Within Continental USA
Tel: 1(800)272 7737; Fax: 1(800)374 3401
Outside Continental USA
Tel: (561)994 0555; Fax: (561)361 6018
E-mail: orders@crcpress.com

Book orders in the rest of the world
Paul Abrahams
Tel: +44 207 017 4036
Email: bookorders@informa.com

Composition by C&M Digitals (P) Ltd, Chennai, India
Printed and bound in India by Replika Press Pvt Ltd

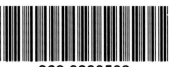

369 0280502

This book is due for return on or before the last date shown below.

A L

E
S

Contents

Dedication

Eleni Symeou, my trusted
secretary for over 20 years

Introduction

Angina pectoris is a common symptom, usually reflecting obstructive coronary artery disease (CAD). As the location and extent of the coronary disease, along with the quality of left ventricular (LV) function, determine prognosis it is important to make an accurate diagnosis as soon as possible. Management is designed not only to relieve symptoms and thereby improve the quality of life, but also, by appropriately timed non-invasive and invasive investigations, to identify those at most risk so that we can select optimal therapy which will also lengthen life.

The aims of treatment are therefore:

- to reduce or abolish symptoms thereby improving quality of life
- to improve prognosis by preventing myocardial infarction and death
- preferably both of the above

This handbook is meant to be practical and to help answer the following questions:

- is it angina?
- how should I treat it?
- who should be referred?
- what tests are needed and when?
- what is the place of drugs, angioplasty and surgery?

This fourth edition has been revised and expanded with regard to the increasing importance of managing hyperlipidaemia, diagnosing and treating CAD in women and the elderly, and managing chest pain in the presence of normal coronary arteries. In addition, the roles of medicine, percutaneous coronary intervention (PCI) and coronary artery bypass grafting (CABG) have been updated and compared.

The main focus of this book is on the evaluation and management of stable angina pectoris. Other manifestations of angina are summarized and brief guidelines on management provided.

Background

Incidence and prevalence

Definitions

Diagnosis of chest pain

Stable angina: clinical evaluation

Investigations

Incidence and prevalence

In the UK about 5% of men and 4% of women have or have had angina. Each year in the UK alone, 320 000 people consult for angina and 340 000 experience myocardial infarcts.

CAD is an equal opportunity killer affecting postmenopausal and premenopausal women as well as men. Among women, deaths from ischaemic heart disease (IHD) are seven times more common than deaths from breast cancer (Table 1) and four times more common than deaths from lung cancer.

In both sexes the prevalence of angina increases with age. Between 45 and 54 years of age, 2–5% of men and 0.1–1% of women have angina but this rises to 11–20% of men and 10–15% of women aged between 65 and 74 years. Above 75 years of age, the prevalence is the same for men and women, at 1 in 3. In Europe where CAD is common, approximately 20 000 to 40 000 per 1 million of the population (men and women) have angina, and half of these are significantly limited as a consequence.

- 1 in 8 men and 1 in 16 women aged 40–44 years have CAD
- 1 in 6 men and 1 in 12 women aged 45–50 years have CAD
- 1 in 5 men and 1 in 9 women aged 45–64 years have CAD
- 1 in 3 men and women aged over 65 years have some form of cardiovascular disease, including angina

Though overall death rates from cardiovascular disease are declining (Figure 1), the number of men and women living with cardiovascular disease is increasing. As women and men are living longer the burden of cardiovascular disease will not decrease. Maintaining quality of life with optimal therapy will therefore be of increasing importance.

Cardiovascular disease is therefore a major concern for women and men and the leading cause of death for both. It is not a matter of whether women can develop CAD—but when.

It is important that both doctors and other healthcare professionals (and women) become aware of the possibility of women developing CAD and that the potential for ischaemia is treated as vigorously in women as in men.

Prevalence is defined as the number of existing cases in the population. Incidence is the number of new cases in a specific period of time.

Table 1   *Causes of death in men and women*

Disease	Men (%)	Women (%)
CAD	21	23
Stroke	11	18
Other CVD	11	15
Cancer	21	18 (breast 3)
Respiratory	8	6
Injuries/poisoning	12	4
Other	16	16

World Health Organization figures for Europe 2004. (www.who.int/whosis)
CAD, coronary artery disease; CVD, cardiovascular disease.

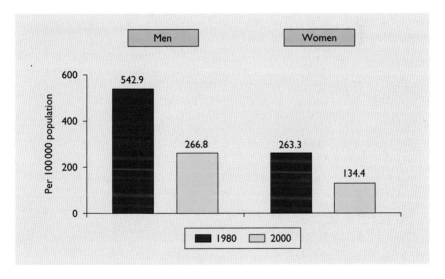

Figure 1   *Age-adjusted death rate for coronary heart disease: 1980–2000. (Ford et al. N. Engl J. Med. 2007; 356: 2388–98.)*

Cost

The indirect costs of CAD are significant, with 12% of the working days that are lost in the UK through sickness being due to CAD—about £1.8 billion annually in lost earnings. The annual direct cost to the NHS is estimated at £3500 million. In the USA, the annual cost is approximately $117 billion.

Age

As the population ages and more people survive heart attacks, the incidence of angina as a manifestation of CAD will increase. In addition, by educating the public and increasing awareness of CAD there should be an increasing workload as people come forward and the need for precise investigation and diagnosis will become even more important.

- Coronary artery disease is the leading cause of death in men and women
- Angina is common and will become more common as the population is ageing
- Effective evidence-based strategies for diagnosis, investigation and treatment are essential

Definitions

Stable angina

Stable angina is ischaemic cardiac pain, which may be perceived in many ways (Table 2), that is brought on by effort and relieved by rest. It will have been present for several weeks or longer. It is precipitated by predictable factors and relieved promptly by rest and/or sublingual nitrates. It will not have worsened recently in terms of severity of attacks, increasing frequency of attacks or attacks at rest (Table 3).

Table 2   *Characteristics of cardiac pain*

Typical
Tightness
Pressure
Weight
Constriction
Ache
Dull
Squeezing feeling
Crushing
'Like a band'
Breathless (tightness)
Retrosternal
Precipitated by exertion or emotion
Promptly relieved by rest of glyceryl trinitrate
Atypical
Sharp (not severe)
Knife-like
Stabbing
'Like a stitch'
'Like a needle'
Pricking feeling

(Continued)

Table 2 *Continued*

Shooting

Can walk around with it

Continuous: 'it's there all day'

Located in left chest, abdomen, back or arm in absence of mid-chest pain

Unrelated to exercise

Not relieved by rest or glyceryl trinitrate

Relieved by antacids; characterized by palpitations without chest pain

Women

At rest

During sleep

Stress

Jaw, teeth, arms, neck, shoulders, back, abdomen

Table 3 *The widely used subjective grading of angina of effort by the Canadian Cardiovascular Society*

Grading of angina of effort
1. 'Ordinary physical activity does not cause angina': this includes walking and climbing stairs. Angina occurs with strenuous or rapid or prolonged exertion at work or recreation.
2. 'Slight limitation of ordinary activity': this includes walking or climbing stairs rapidly, walking uphill, walking or climbing stairs after meals, or in the cold, or in wind, or under emotional stress, or only during the few hours after awakening; walking more than two blocks[†] on the level and climbing more than one flight of ordinary stairs at a normal pace and in normal conditions.
3. 'Marked limitation of ordinary physical activity': this includes walking one to two blocks[†] on the level and climbing one flight of stairs in normal conditions and at normal pace.
4. 'Inability to carry on any physical activity without discomfort—angina syndrome may be present at rest'.

[†] One block equals 100–200 metres.

Angina is a clinical diagnosis based on the doctor's interpretation of the patient's story. A good history needs no confirmatory tests, but tests will be needed to evaluate risk and optimize management.

Unstable angina

The term 'unstable angina' describes a clinical presentation between stable angina and myocardial infarction (MI); it may move in either direction. Clinically the presentation can be divided into three groups:

- effort angina of recent onset (less than 1 month) at a low workload (22.5–45 metres walking on the flat)—no previous angina
- changing pattern of angina with stable angina increasing in frequency and/or severity for no obvious reason
- angina at rest (up to 20 minutes)

Only one criterion is required for the diagnosis, but two or three may be present.

Other names for unstable angina include the intermediate coronary syndrome, pre-infarction angina, crescendo angina, acute coronary sufficiency and accelerated angina. It is included now in the umbrella term 'acute coronary syndrome'.

Diagnosis of chest pain

There are many causes of chest pain. Clinically, we are concerned with differentiating angina from chest wall pain, oesophageal pain or functional pain that may be linked to hyperventilation. Since angina is such an important clinical diagnosis, it is essential to rule it in or out accurately. If in doubt, further evaluation (e.g. by exercise testing) is strongly advised.

Nature of the pain

Ischaemic pain can be defined by asking the following questions:

- site—where is the pain?
- radiation—where does it go?
- character—what does it feel like?
- causes—what brings it on?
- relief—what do you do when you have the pain; do you have to slow down or stop?

Site

The site of pain may be retrosternal: this can be localized but is more usually spread across the chest.

The patient may place his or her hand across the chest (Figure 2) or clench the fist (Figure 3), emphasizing the squeezing constriction that is sometimes felt.

The pain is only very rarely localized (Figure 4)—this is usually muscular chest wall pain.

Radiation

Pain usually radiates out from the chest rather than into the chest. Presentation in referral sites only is unusual but can be dangerous, particularly if there is severe epigastric pain, which may lead to an inappropriate gastroscopy or laparotomy (Table 4).

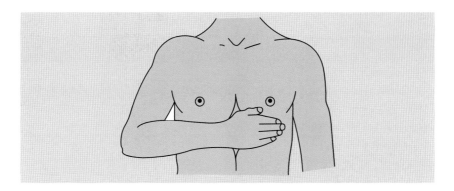

Figure 2 *The patient may draw the flat of his hand across the chest.*

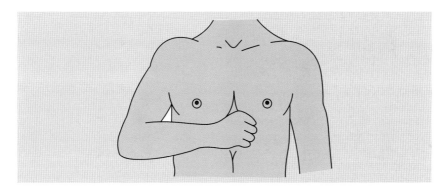

Figure 3 *Clenched fist in the centre (Levine's sign) illustrating the constriction or tightness felt.*

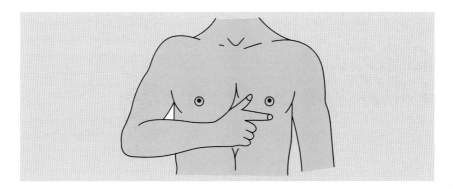

Figure 4 *The patient almost never points to the pain as if it is localized.*

Table 4   Sites of anginal pain in 150 successive ambulatory patients

Location of pain	Sole involvement (per cent)	Partial involvement (per cent)
Anterior chest	34.0	96.0
Left arm (upper)	0.7	30.7
Left arm (lower)	1.3	29.3
Right arm (upper)	0	10.0
Right arm (lower)	0	13.3
Back	0.7	16.7
Epigastrium	0.7	3.3
Forehead	0	6.0
Neck	2.0	22.0
Chin and perioral area	0	8.7

The commonest sites are shown in Figure 5. They include:

- neck and throat—patients present with a 'choking', 'strangling' or 'suffocating' feeling
- jaw—'toothache', 'dentures a problem'
- left arm, right arm or both—pain is usually felt down the inside of the arm under the axilla to the inner two fingers (muscular pain usually runs over the shoulder and down the outside of the arm)
- abdomen—'indigestion'
- back—'arthritis'
- site of previous injury (e.g. fractured arm, severe spondylosis, carious tooth)

Anyone presenting with epigastric pain who is over 40 years of age and at cardiac risk (e.g. smoker, hypertensive, male, diabetic) should have an electrocardiogram (ECG) and there should be a high index of suspicion for a cardiac cause, even if the story strongly suggests a gastric problem.

Character

The sensation may be so mild that it is often dismissed by the patient as an ache or 'indigestion' rather than a pain. The commonest features are summarized in Table 2. The following are of note:

- tightness is often perceived as breathlessness
- the pain usually builds up rather than being maximal at its onset
- sharp, knife-like pain of sudden onset is not cardiac

12

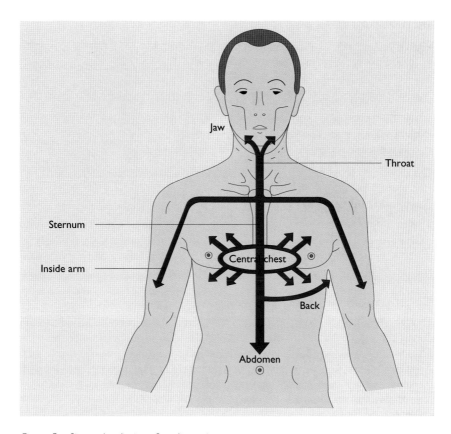

Figure 5 *Site and radiation of cardiac pain.*

- beware local dialects—for example 'sharp' can sometimes mean 'severe' not 'knife-like'
- watch the patient's hands as he or she talks—they often tell the story for the patient (Figures 2–4)
- if the patient is breathless, ask what this means—is it a tightness or a winded feeling?

Causes

Angina is brought on by an increase in oxygen demand that cannot be met by supply. It usually lasts longer than 15 seconds and less than 15 minutes, the average being 3 minutes or less. With a supply and demand problem caused by obstructive CAD, any factor that increases heart rate (i.e. demand) at the expense of supply (shorter diastole—the coronaries fill in diastole) can induce pain.

13

The commonest causes are:

- exertion: inclines, and stairs in particular
- emotion: especially anger and anxiety
- a large meal: cardiac output rises 20%
- temperature change
- windy weather
- exciting programmes on TV: so-called 'match of the day' angina
- vivid dreams: particularly if these are frightening
- sexual intercourse: especially if this is extramarital or casual

The above may be additive (e.g. walking the dog in windy weather after a meal).

Postprandial angina

This is angina within 30 minutes of a meal. It appears to be a marker of severity of disease and is more often associated with unstable angina. Particularly in patients with a previous myocardial infarct, it suggests severe coronary disease and should serve as an indication for early angiography.

Chest pain in women

Though chest pain in women is common, it is often atypical and difficult to pin down (Table 2). With the lower prevalence of disease in younger women, both the history and exercise ECGs are more likely to be false positive for CAD. Approximately 40% of women with chest pain have normal coronary arteries with the only factor consistently predicting CAD being diabetes. In spite of normal coronary arteries, an appreciable number of women continue to experience symptoms that often prove difficult to manage (see page 75). Where symptoms are atypical or minimal and/or where doubts exist, i.e. where the doctor cannot say whether the patient is normal or not, further tests are required.

Relief

Slowing the heart rate by rest or relaxation will reduce demand. For example, the patient may walk slowly or sit down. Glyceryl trinitrate (GTN) relieves pain by vasodilatation, reducing demand. Relief is rapid—usually in less than 10 minutes.

Pain relieved previously by GTN which now lengthens to 30 minutes may reflect unstable angina or infarction. GTN may modify but not relieve this pain.

Unstable angina

Unstable angina may be new or worsening angina. Angina is noted at rest or minimal activity, and exercise tolerance may be suddenly and dramatically reduced.

It is still usually relieved by GTN (see page 78).

Variant angina

Variant angina is also known as Prinzmetal's angina. It is caused by spasm on a fixed coronary lesion or occasionally by spasm when the coronary arteries are normal. It occurs:

- usually at rest
- in response to cold
- rarely on exercise
- at a consistent time of day—usually night or early morning
- often with the sensation of palpitation

The presence of ST elevation on an ECG during ischaemia separates variant angina from the more usual ST depression seen in other forms of angina.

Uncommon angina presentations

'Second wind angina' is the ability to walk off the pain, especially if the exercise is pleasurable (e.g. golf). This may be due to ischaemic preconditioning.

'Tobacco angina' is pain on smoking cigarettes or, rarely, cigars.

In angina decubitus, the pain is worse when the patient lies down in bed. This is rare: perhaps dreams, or a cold bedroom or cold sheets are the cause (it is not due to syphilis, as was originally taught).

Angina with syncope, which is more common in the elderly, points to severe CAD.

Pain from myocardial infarction

Pain from myocardial infarction lasts longer than angina—usually over 30 minutes—and is severe and retrosternal. It is characterized by pallor, perspiration, nausea and vomiting.

The pain is not relieved by GTN but it may be modified.

Differential diagnosis

From the cardiac point of view there are two important differential diagnoses: acute pericarditis and dissecting aortic aneurysm. Non-cardiac causes of chest pain include pain secondary to pulmonary disease, gastrointestinal problems, musculoskeletal pain and functional chest pain (Table 5).

As well as excluding non-cardiac causes of chest pain the doctor must remember that coexisting pathologies may be present, especially in older patients (e.g. hiatus hernia and angina), so it is important to entertain the possibility of one or more chest pain aetiologies being present at the same time.

Table 5   *Some differential features of chest pain*

Differential diagnosis
Oesophageal
Not usually exertional. Rarely radiates to left arm. Worse when lying flat or after a large meal. Relieved by belching, standing, antacids but also occasionally by GTN and calcium antagonists. May coexist with angina.
Pericarditis
Sharp pain worse on inspiration and lying flat. Relieved by shallow breathing and standing. Often pyrexial. Rub may be audible.
Pulmonary
Pleuritic pain, worse with breathing, often localized. Frequent cough or haemoptysis. Rub audible.
Musculoskeletal
Positional, localized, reproduced by pressure. Sharp, suddenly severe. May be tightness due to pectoral spasm. May be deep to the breast in women. Often pointed to with one or two fingers.
Functional
Hyperventilation. Patient easily breathless, frequent sighs, anxious, often young woman Musculoskeletal pain may be associated.
Mitral valve prolapse
Mostly atypical but some typical pains and more common in younger women who may also hyperventilate. Frequently pain after exercise when fatigued.
Dissecting aortic aneurysm
Very severe pain to the back. At its most severe at its onset. May radiate to the lower abdomen, thighs and hips. Not affected by posture.

Practical points

- Use the key questions to help make the diagnosis
- Angina is usually brought on by effort and relieved by rest, and most patients have a typical history. Women, however, tend to have more atypical features
- When the story is not clear, ask the patient to imagine that he or she is walking up an incline and to describe what happens
- Relatives and friends can often provide helpful additional information

Stable angina: clinical evaluation

Aetiology

Obstructive CAD is the commonest cause of angina pectoris. Other conditions with or without coexistent CAD can independently cause angina or exacerbate angina that is due to underlying CAD. These conditions include:

- coronary spasm: this usually occurs as rest pain
- aortic stenosis: the patient is usually over 60 years of age
- aortic incompetence: the patient is usually over 60 years of age
- left ventricular hypertrophy: this occurs with hypertension and cardiomyopathy. Hypertrophic cardiomyopathy can present at any age
- anaemia
- thyrotoxicosis
- rapid or slow arrhythmias: these occur particularly in the elderly (atrial fibrillation)
- severe mitral stenosis: a very rare cause
- primary pulmonary hypertension: this is also very rare

Examination

Usually no abnormality is found on clinical examination. Careful assessment may identify diagnostic clues:

- nicotine-stained fingers or smell of tobacco
- anaemia
- premature arcus senilis in a patient less than 40 years old
- xanthomas on the hands, elbows, knees or ankles, which indicate familial hyper-cholesterolaemia
- xanthelasma is surprisingly non-specific

The commonest auscultatory finding is a fourth heart sound (listen with the bell at the apex)—this reflects reduced ventricular compliance. The commonest overall finding is hypertension. Check for:

- murmurs, which may be a sign of aortic and mitral valve disease
- apical dyskinesia, indicating left ventricular ischaemia or infarction
- hypertension
- isolated systolic hypertension: think also of aortic regurgitation

- carotid or femoral bruits
- peripheral pulses, which may be absent especially in those with diabetes or in heavy smokers
- signs of diabetes

A practical checklist is given in Table 6.

Table 6 Examination checklist

Sign	Location	Comment
Xanthoma	Hands, elbows, knees	Hyperlipidaemia
Xanthelasma	Eyelids	Non-specific
Arcus senilis	Eyes	Non-specific over 40 years of age
Fourth heart sound	Apex (turn to left side)	Reduced ventricular compliance
Immediate diastolic murmur	Third or fourth left intercostal space, patient leaning forward	Aortic incompetence
Ejection systolic murmur	Apex, second right intercostal space, neck	Aortic stenosis
Late or pansystolic murmur	Apex to axilla	Mitral regurgitation
Bruits	Both carotid and femoral arteries	Peripheral arterial disease

Investigations

Patients with severe symptoms in spite of medical therapy have selected themselves for further investigations with a view to angioplasty (percutaneous coronary intervention, PCI) or surgery (coronary artery bypass grafting, CABG). Unfortunately those with mild symptoms may have severe and prognostically important CAD and we need to identify them.

Three questions therefore need to be answered:

- Who is at risk?
- How do we identify him or her?
- Can we modify the risk?

However, before embarking on a series of investigations to try to identify who is at risk, we need to know the degree of risk and the evidence that one form of therapy above another will reduce the risk. From this knowledge will come guidelines on referral.

Natural history

Patients with stable angina have a good prognosis whatever we do. Each year, 2–3% will die and a similar number will suffer from non-fatal myocardial infarction. However, some patients are more at risk of cardiac events than others. These high-risk patients are those with:

- significant left ventricular dysfunction
- left main stem disease (> 50% stenosis)
- severe three-vessel CAD (> 70% proximal stenoses)
- > 70% two-vessel disease, including proximal left anterior descending disease

It is important to identify those at risk and it is vital, once someone at risk is identified, that we have evidence of benefit from one strategy of care above others. This is not so straightforward as it seems because many of the trials comparing treatments are old and overall management has changed significantly.

There are two aims of treatment:

- to relieve symptoms
- to improve prognosis

Symptom relief

There is clear evidence of symptomatic benefit from drug therapy, PCI and CABG.

There is no evidence in the absence of a proven prognostic benefit that PCI or CABG should be first-choice therapy for symptom relief.

- The primary symptomatic treatment of stable angina is medical, and optimal medical therapy includes general advice, risk factor reduction and specific antianginal agents

Improving prognosis—who is at risk?

Certain medical treatments have been shown to improve prognosis:

- beta-blockers post-infarction
- lipid-lowering drugs—statins
- aspirin
- angiotensin-converting enzyme (ACE) inhibitors with a coexisting history of MI, hypertension, LV dysfunction (ejection fraction [EF] <40%), diabetes or impaired renal function.

CABG has been shown to improve prognosis for some patients when compared with medical therapy or PCI. CABG is recommended prognostically when there is:

- left main stem disease or its equivalent (severe stenosis of ostial/proximal left anterior descending and circumflex arteries)
- three-vessel CAD with impaired LV function (EF < 30%) or early or extensive ischaemia on non-invasive testing
- disease of the proximal left anterior descending artery as part of two-vessel CAD with reversible ischaemia on non-invasive testing

Relieving symptoms
Comparing medicine, PCI and CABG

Many trials exist comparing the three strategies but most have been outdated by improvements in drug therapy and technology. In general PCI has not been demonstrated to improve survival in patients with stable angina when compared with optimal medical therapy. The COURAGE trial compared PCI plus optimal medical therapy ($n = 1149$) with optimal medical therapy alone ($n = 1138$) in men and women with stable angina. PCI did not reduce the risk of death, MI or other major cardiovascular events when added to optimal medical therapy. PCI was initially more effective in relieving anginal symptoms but this benefit decreased over time so that after five years follow-up there was no difference between optimal medical therapy alone and PCI plus medical therapy (Boden 2007).

The 5-year follow-up of the Medicine, Angioplasty or Surgery Study (MASS II) compared 611 patients with stable angina, 203 of whom underwent CABG, 205 PCI and 203 medical therapy. There was no difference in cardiac-related death or overall mortality between all three groups. All had preserved LV function and left main CAD was excluded. The authors concluded that PCI and CABG should be reserved for those symptomatic in spite of medical therapy in the presence of low-risk anatomy (Hueb).

After comprehensively reviewing comparative studies and after excluding prognostically high-risk anatomy, the European Society of Cardiology recommended intervention with revascularization for the relief of symptoms in spite of optimal medical therapy: PCI or CABG to be determined by anatomic suitability and operator experience/success rates. Medical therapy to optimize risk reduction will need to be continued post PCI or CABG (Fox).

To summarize

- Stable angina has a low event rate so there is time to optimize management
- Medical therapy to relieve symptoms and reduce risk should be initiated at diagnosis
- Non-invasive testing should be employed to look for high-risk cases
- PCI is effective in relieving pain that persists in spite of medical therapy
- PCI is not prognostically indicated
- CABG relieves pain and also improves prognosis in high-risk patients

Identifying those at risk

The only absolute way to evaluate CAD is by angiography. Where practical, those below 50 years of age should undergo this procedure because decisions made are for 20–30 years and should be based on the fullest possible information. Resources may limit this arbitrary age level to 40 years of age. However, cardiac computed tomography (page 27) may become the screening test of choice.

Electrocardiography

The resting ECG is the most widely applied test in the evaluation of angina pectoris. It is not a substitute for a good clinical history and clinical judgement. It may

Boden WE, O'Rourke RA, Teo KK et al. Optimal medical therapy with or without PCI for stable coronary disease. N Engl J Med 2007; 356: 1503–16.

Hueb W, Lopes NH, Gersh BJ et al. Five year follow-up of the Medicine, Angioplasty, or Surgery Study (MASS II). Circulation 2007; 115: 1082–9.

Fox K, Garcia MAA, Ardissino D et al. Guidelines on the management of stable angina pectoris. Eur Heart J 2006; 27: 1341–81.

be normal in up to 50% of patients with angina, even in the presence of severe symptoms. A normal ECG therefore does not rule out CAD but it does suggest good left ventricular function. An abnormal resting ECG identifies a patient group at higher risk of death and myocardial infarction—changes may be non-specific ST depression or T-wave inversion, but previous infarction may also be identified. Left bundle branch block suggests left ventricular impairment and possibly multivessel CAD. In addition, the ECG may identify left ventricular hypertrophy or arrhythmias. Old ECG traces should be reviewed if they are available, since changes from normal to abnormal or vice versa may identify ischaemic events, new or old.

- A normal ECG does not rule out CAD

Exercise ECG

The accuracy of an exercise test depends on the prevalence of the disease in the study group. Applied to young women (aged 30–39 years) who rarely have CAD, a negative test at a good workload will have a 99% accuracy in ruling out CAD but a positive test will have an 80% chance of being falsely positive. Applying the test to a group of men with a high probability of CAD increases its accuracy significantly—the sensitivity averages 70% and the specificity 90%, whereas in women the sensitivity averages 61% and the specificity 69%. The sensitivity relates to patients with disease; the specificity excludes those without disease.

- Exercise testing is less accurate in women than in men

Symptom-related treadmill exercise ECGs in the absence of cardioactive drugs that can modify the ST segment are the most accurate. Indications are:

- to clarify the diagnosis where doubts exist—no age barrier if in good overall health
- to identify those at risk up to 70 years of age
- to objectively assess disability
- to monitor progress and effect of therapy
- to aid rehabilitation

Exercise testing with medical supervision is safe, with a complication rate of ventricular fibrillation of 1 in 5000, but there are contraindications, which are outlined below.

Contraindications to exercise testing

Absolute contraindications

- Acute myocardial infarction (within 7 days)
- Unstable angina

- Uncontrolled cardiac arrhythmias causing symptoms or haemodynamic compromise
- Severe aortic stenosis
- Uncontrolled heart failure
- Acute pulmonary embolus or pulmonary infarction
- Myocarditis or pericarditis
- Aortic dissection
- Severe arterial hypertension (systolic blood pressure > 200 mmHg and/or diastolic blood pressure > 110 mmHg)

Relative contraindications

- Left main coronary stenosis
- Moderate stenotic valvular heart disease
- Tachyarrhythmias or bradyarrhythmias
- Hypertrophic cardiomyopathy

Endpoints identifying high risk are:

- significant ST depression (> 1 mm), usually with pain
- slow ST recovery to normal (5 minutes or longer)
- fall in systolic blood pressure (> 20 mmHg), reflecting a fall in cardiac output
- rise in diastolic blood pressure (> 15 mmHg); a fall in output causes reflex vasoconstriction
- angina with or without ST changes at a low workload (< 6 minutes)
- dangerous arrhythmias (e.g. ventricular tachycardia)
- ST depression (> 3 mm) without pain

Endpoints signifying low risk are:

- able to exercise to stage 3 (over 9 minutes) or beyond of the Bruce treadmill protocol with no ST changes
- able to achieve stage 4 (12 minutes) or beyond despite ST changes

The Duke treadmill score is a validated risk score combining exercise time, ST deviation and angina during exercise. The score is the exercise time in minutes minus 5 times the ST deviation in millimetres, 4 times the angina index (0 if no angina, 1 angina occurs, 2 angina stops the test). A score of 5 and above is low risk (annual mortality 0.25%); between 4 and −10 is intermediate risk (annual mortality 1.25%); and a score of −11 or below represents high risk (annual mortality 5.25%).

The ST segment can be modified by digoxin and beta-blockers, which should be discontinued if it is clinically safe to do so (digoxin 7 days before the test, beta-blockers 48 hours before the test). Nitrates and calcium antagonists should not be taken on the day of the test.

Exercise test terminology is as follows:

'True positive'	positive exercise test, proven CAD
'True negative'	negative exercise test, normal coronaries
'False positive'	positive test, normal arteries
'False negative'	negative test, proven CAD
'Sensitivity' (%)	$\dfrac{\text{true positive}}{\text{true negatives} + \text{false negatives}} \times 100$
'Specificity' (%)	$\dfrac{\text{true negatives}}{\text{true nagatives} + \text{false positive}} \times 100$
'Predictive accuracy' (%)	$\dfrac{\text{true positives}}{\text{true positives} + \text{false positives}} \times 100$

Thus, 'sensitivity' is the percentage of patients with CAD who have an abnormal exercise ECG, 'specificity' is the percentage of negative tests in patients without CAD and 'predictive accuracy' is the percentage of positive tests that are truly positive.

Thus, sensitivity detects patients with disease and specificity excludes those without disease:

- angina and ST depression > 1 mm gives a predictive accuracy of 90% for CAD
- ST depression > 2 mm is virtually diagnostic for CAD in the absence of left ventricular hypertrophy
- ST depression > 1 mm and no pain has a predictive value of 70% for CAD; and ST depression > 2 mm has a predictive value of 90% for CAD
- false-positive tests are more common in women
- overall sensitivity averages 68%; overall specificity averages 77%

Problem areas exist: with left bundle branch block, one cannot interpret the ECG; there may be physical limitation (e.g. arthritis) or a lack of coordination (so the patient cannot exercise properly).

- Overall, the exercise ECG is a simple, safe and inexpensive investigation that provides extremely useful information to aid diagnosis and management

Ambulatory ECGs

Ambulatory ECGs for 24–48 hours add little to the management of stable angina since they are less accurate than exercise ECGs in predicting risk. They are unhelpful with left bundle branch block but they can be useful in evaluating pain when physical limitation prohibits exercise testing, when chest pain occurs at night or when chest pain is linked to arrhythmias.

Ambulatory monitoring has also identified ST changes in the absence of symptoms—*silent myocardial ischaemia*. This may occur in patients with CAD who never have angina (type 1) or in those who do experience angina but who have both painful and painless ischaemia (type 2).

Management is controversial but, when risk is being assessed, silent ischaemia on a treadmill ECG does predict an adverse outcome. Ambulatory monitoring is less accurate, however, and should be reserved for selected patients who have proven ischaemic heart disease (e.g. previous infarction) and no confusing factors such as left bundle branch block, left ventricular hypertrophy or strain or digoxin therapy. The effect of drug therapy or intervention can be evaluated by serial monitoring.

Nuclear imaging

Nuclear scanning has a helpful role in addition to exercise ECG. It needs specialized equipment and is more expensive, but it is useful in the presence of left bundle branch block, when routine exercise tests are non-diagnostic or borderline, or when cardiovascular stress is limited by poor exercise ability.

Thallium-201 is taken up by the perfused myocardium. Note that:

- infarction is a 'cold' area that fails to fill in
- exercise may cause a cold area that fills in later: this is a sign of reversible ischaemia
- partial filling suggests ischaemia adjacent to infarction

Thallium imaging is superior to exercise testing for the diagnosis of CAD. It has a sensitivity of 85–90% (versus 68%) and a specificity of 70–75% (versus 77%) using exercise and 83–94% and 64–90% with pharmacological stress (e.g. dobutamine). In some studies it has been shown to predict subsequent cardiac events and prognosis more accurately, with event rates related exponentially and independently to both the extent and the severity of reversible ischaemia. It is, however, more expensive and requires specialized equipment, and the more accurate tomographic techniques (single-photon emission computed tomography; SPECT) are technically demanding—its role remains valuable but limited. It can be helpful in relating the coronary anatomy to the extent of ischaemia when planning angioplasty or CABG. A normal thallium scan has a very low event rate—less than 1% per year—and can be regarded as very reassuring, particularly in the presence of atypical chest pain and equivocal exercise ECGs whereas abnormal scans increase the risk nine-fold.

Low-cost, low-radiation, generator-produced and easily available radiopharmaceuticals (e.g. ^{99m}technetium sestamibi) offer better imaging than and advantages over thallium, since they need less specialized facilities (i.e. it has a wider applicability) and there is evidence that SPECT sestamibi (i.e. three-dimensional views) reduces the rate of false positives and improves the specificity for the detection of CAD.

However, although myocardial perfusion imagery, particularly SPECT, is the most important aspect of nuclear cardiology, cost will limit its applicability. For the present it is helpful:

- when there is left bundle branch block, paced rhythm or Wolff–Parkinson–White syndrome which prevent accurate ECG interpretation during exercise alone
- when the functional significance of the established CAD is uncertain
- when exercise stress is not possible (e.g. in peripheral vascular disease or arthritis)
- when the exercise ECG is equivocal
- when ischaemic left ventricular dysfunction is present and the degree of reversibility is questioned
- to assess the success of CABG or PTCA, particularly if atypical symptoms persist

Thallium imaging is less accurate in women, owing to breast artefact (78% sensitivity, 64% specificity).

Those who cannot exercise may have ischaemia induced by dipyridamole, dobutamine or adenosine.

Positron emission tomography

Positron emission tomography (PET) is an expensive technique that uses positron emitters with very short half-lives as tracers. PET requires both an on-site cyclotron (for the production of the tracers) and radiochemistry facilities. The technique involves radiation and is expensive and slow, but it does provide the opportunity of measuring regional blood flow accurately. In clinical practice it can identify hibernating myocardium in patients in whom prognosis would be improved by intervention and improved ventricular function. Hibernating myocardium is still viable but unable to function owing to severely limited blood supply. The advantage over thallium is at best marginal and is unlikely to justify anything other than highly selected and research use. However, in women, PET appears to be a very accurate diagnostic test with false-positive and false-negative rates as low as 5–10%, but cost limits its use.

Echocardiography

Echocardiography at rest

This provides a useful, non-invasive assessment of left ventricular function and hypertrophy and a means of clarifying the significance of murmurs. Echocardiography may visualize the left main stem but otherwise does not provide pictures of the coronary arteries. It may complement exercise testing by identifying poor left ventricular function as a cause for a poor ability to exercise and thereby dictate risk, the need for further investigation and the need for prognostically indicated drugs such as ACE inhibitors. The 12-year survival with an EF of > 50% is 73% compared with an EF of 35–49% (54% survival) and an EF of < 35% (21% survival).

Stress echocardiography

This technique also utilizes exercise or pharmacology to induce ischaemia. However, up to 20% of patients who need their chest pain evaluated cannot adequately exercise on a treadmill or bicycle. Dobutamine stress echocardiography has been shown to be a valuable alternative for them. Intravenous dobutamine is gradually increased in dosage, increasing heart rate in a similar way to conventional exercise testing. Continuous ECG and echocardiographic monitoring is performed. Normal myocardium increases in movement and thickening, whereas ischaemic myocardium shows reduced thickening and transient movement abnormalities. Hibernating myocardium can also be assessed—this is myocardium that appears to be irreversibly damaged but that may demonstrate viability and therefore be a candidate for revascularization.

- Compared with a conventional exercise ECG, exercise stress echo is a more accurate diagnostic test in women, with an 84–85% sensitivity and 84–86% specificity

Echocardiograms are cheap, safe, reproducible and repeatable and may therefore be of more clinical benefit than radionuclide studies. The place of stress echocardiography is similar to that of nuclear studies as detailed above—it is employed:

- when there is left bundle branch block
- when conventional exercise is not possible

- to assess the degree of ischaemic left ventricular dysfunction
- to assess the functional significance of documented CAD on left ventricular performance
- to judge the value of intervention
- when exercise ECGs are equivocal in women

Computed tomography

Electron-beam computed tomography detects coronary artery calcification which is part of the atherosclerotic process. The extent of calcification increases the likelihood of a non-fatal MI or cardiac death over 5–7 years.

Multi-detector computed tomography or multislice CT is the most promising technique for the non-invasive imaging of the coronary arteries. Sensitivity and specificity using 64-slice detector scanners is 90–94% and 95–97%, respectively, with an important negative predictive value of 93–99%.

Due to a radiation dose similar to that of invasive coronary angiography, the technique is currently recommended for patients with a low probability of CAD and for those at high risk or with an equivocal result on conventional exercise or stress imaging.

However, this exciting technique is likely to increase in use as its value prognostically is defined.

Magnetic resonance arteriography

A non-invasive test without X-ray exposure. Not yet in routine clinical practice for stable angina. First data domonstrates that patients with a negative magnetic resonanance scan have an excellent prognosis.

Coronary angiography

Coronary angiography is currently the definitive diagnostic test: it accurately assesses the anatomy. A stenosis is significant when the lumen is narrow by 70% or more or 50% in the left main coronary artery. It may not identify minor plaque disease in contrast to computed tomography.

Day-case procedures are increasingly employed. Important complications occur in just under 1% of patients, with death in 0.11%. These figures include high-risk cases, so routine procedures will be at lower risk.

Coronary anatomy is shown in Figure 6.

Figure 7 summarizes the investigative approach. This is equivalent to 3000 exercise tests and 700–1000 angiograms per million of the population per year.

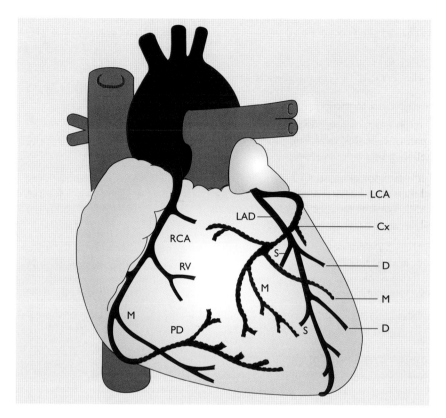

Figure 6 *Schematic chart of the major coronary arteries. The posterior descending (PD) may arise from the right coronary artery (RCA, right dominant artery) or circumflex artery (Cx, left dominant artery). D, diagonal artery; LAD, left anterior descending artery; LCA, left coronary artery; M, marginal branches; RV, branch to the right ventricle; S, septal branch. Dotted arteries indicate that these are on the posterior side of the heart.*

Angiography is indicated:

- when symptoms are severe in spite of optimal medical therapy—there is no age barrier for patients in good overall health
- when there is evidence of increased risk, irrespective of symptoms
- survivors of cardiac arrest
- when angina recurs after PCI or CABG
- when the diagnosis needs to be clarified and non-invasive tests are equivocal

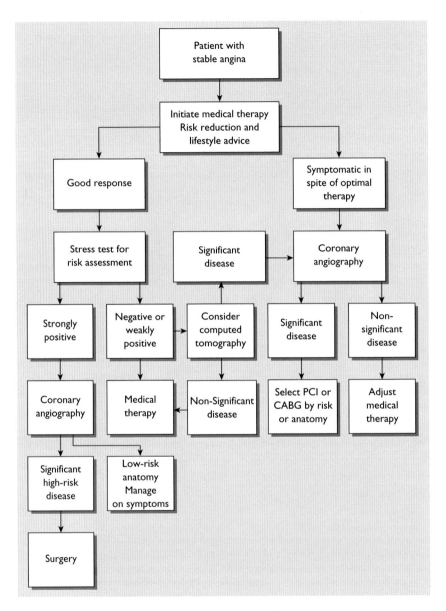

Figure 7 *Investigative approach to the clinical evaluation of the patient with angina pectoris. Nuclear imaging and stress echocardiography complement this algorithm in selected cases.*

Predicting CAD in women

The determinants of CAD in women can be graded. By selecting out major and low-risk groups it becomes possible to maximize the effectiveness of investigations given the overall low prevalence of CAD.

- Major determinants—typical chest pain, especially following menopause, diabetes, peripheral vascular disease
- Intermediate determinants—hypertension, smoking, hyperlipidaemia
- Minor determinants—age over 65 years, obesity, sedentary, family history

A low-risk group would be premenopausal with atypical chest pain and not diabetic; such patients would be estimated to have a less than 20% likelihood of CAD.

A high-risk group with an 80% chance of CAD would include women with two or more major determinants or one major and two or more intermediate or minor determinants.

Most women fall between 20% and 80%, where CAD needs to be ruled in or out. The general algorithm can be modified for women (Figure 8) to enable the targeting of appropriate diagnostic groups, which will increase diagnostic accuracy, reduce cost and enhance clinical practice.

Screening
Lipids

It is now clear that in the presence of established CAD, correcting lipid abnormalities reduces disease progression and may induce disease regression. There is no argument that as a part of secondary prevention all patients should undergo full lipid screening up to 85 years of age, with measurements of total, low-density lipoprotein (LDL) and high-density lipoprotein (HDL) cholesterol, as well as triglycerides. Although, it is debatable that the very elderly need intervention, they can still be used as a means of identifying younger family members who may be at risk and benefit from primary prevention.

Lipid screening is indicated:

- in all patients with established CAD to reduce subsequent ischaemic events
- in families of those with familial hypercholesterolaemia
- in other at-risk groups (e.g. those with diabetes, hypertension or a strong family history of CAD) as both primary and secondary prevention

Exercise ECGs

In the asymptomatic, ECGs are unreliable on exercise (66% false positives). They are, however, useful in those at high risk (e.g. those with familial

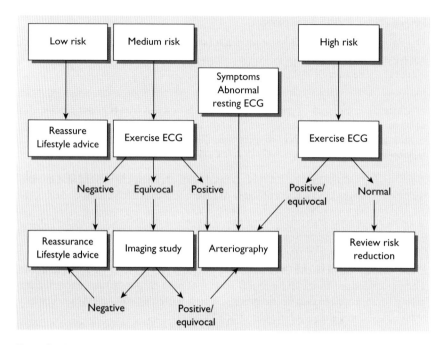

Figure 8 An approach to the management of coronary heart disease in women. Low risk: the estimated risk of CHD is less than 20%; women are likely to be younger, with atypical pain and no risk factors of significance. Moderate risk: risk is 20–80%; a mixture of typical and atypical pain; one major risk factor. High risk: more than 80% likelihood of CHD; typical pain; two major risk factors. Computed tomography could be considered for equivocal cases instead of an imaging study or coronary angiography. (From Wenger NK, Collins P (eds) Women and Heart Disease. London: Taylor & Francis, 2005: 201.)

hypercholesterolaemia—2% of the total population), when an annual review may identify developing CAD.

Otherwise, they are only of value if we are looking for left main stem disease. As this represents only 8% of the angina population, the value of screening the pain-free is extremely limited.

In the UK, the Civil Aviation Authority has rejected exercise ECGs for asymptomatic pilots.

Blood pressure

A check on blood pressure remains the most useful annual check that an asymptomatic person can have.

32

Silent ischaemia

Evaluation has been discussed under ambulatory monitoring (see page 25). Detecting silent ischaemia on exercise testing is a more reliable predictor of CAD than ambulatory monitoring. Thus, the development of silent ischaemia during exercise test screening of those who are asymptomatic but at high risk (e.g. those with hypercholesterolaemia) merits computed tomography or coronary angiography. A high incidence of normal coronary arteries remains.

Referral guidelines

Investigating angina and assessing risk should take into account age as well as symptom limitation.

- Mild symptoms managed medically in the elderly (over 70 years)—no need to refer
- Those who are over 70 years of age who are biologically young and who are symptomatic on medical therapy should proceed to angiography—refer
- Young patients (aged under 50 years) should be managed more aggressively—refer
- Those aged between 50 and 70 years should have their risk status identified—arrange exercise ECG; refer if high risk
- Diagnostic doubts, difficult to interpret and just unsure of the presence or absence of CAD—refer
- Suspect valvular heart disease or left ventricular dysfunction—arrange echocardiogram; refer if significantly abnormal

Management

General management

Drug therapy

Intervention

Refractory angina

Coronary disease in women

Coronary disease in the elderly

General management

The management of angina must take into account both the 'quality' and 'quantity' of life. We need to make people not only feel better but also live longer.

Since stable angina overall has a good prognosis, whatever management is employed, with an annual mortality and non-fatal infarction rate of 2–3% there is time to organize treatment and investigations. Treatment should be initiated in all patients in general practice.

The patient and family need to understand the nature of the problem, what caused it and what can be done to prevent it worsening. Fortunately, most patients benefit from medical therapy but they need to be encouraged to make a major contribution to their own care by correcting any elements of their lifestyle that have contributed to their problem. There is no substitute for a clear personal approach but educational booklets and the internet do provide useful additional information and are always available for reference.

Prevention

The line between primary and secondary prevention is artificial—a man who is asymptomatic on Monday but has a heart attack on Tuesday changes his terminology overnight but not his risk status.

Smoking

Stopping smoking reduces the cardiovascular risk in men and women by 80% over 5 years (Figure 9). It is the cheapest and most cost-effective risk factor modification available. Patients (and their relatives and friends) must be strongly encouraged to stop smoking. Passive smoking should also be avoided. Nicotine patches have been shown to be a safe and effective aid. Alternative drug therapies include buproprion (Zyban) and varenicline (Champix). Support groups and behavioural programmes are also effective.

Obesity

Weight loss may reduce the anginal attack rate, improve physical ability and help with lipid and diabetic control. Abdominal obesity (waist to hip circumference >0.8 in women and >0.9 in men) is more strongly related to CAD risk and mortality. The body mass index (BMI) has largely been replaced by waist circumference as an indication of obesity in clinical practice. In women the measurement

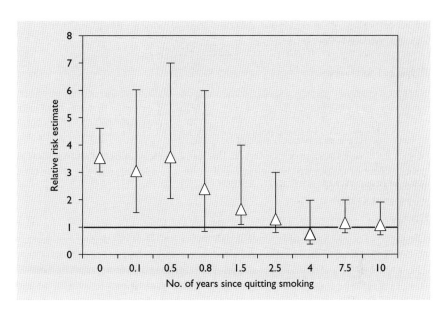

Figure 9 *Rapid impact of smoking cessation on cardiac events in women. Rossenberg et al. N Engl J Med 1990; 322: 213–17.*

should be ≤ 80 cm (31.5 inches), with increased risk 80–87 cm and greater risk ≥ 88 cm. In a man the ideal waist is ≤ 94 cm (37 inches) but lower in Chinese, Japanese and South Asians (90 cm).

Waist size is measured using a tape 1 cm above the navel or midpoint between lowest rib and the iliac crest—patient exhales and the abdomen is relaxed.

Avoiding obesity reduces mortality, with an estimated four-fold reduction in CAD risk. Once a person is obese, it is difficult to lose weight without regular physical activity, which may in turn be restricted by angina. Most people can make sensible dietary changes (eating more vegetables, fruit, fish and poultry, and avoiding excess calories in cakes, biscuits, too much alcohol and oversized portions). Expert help from a dietitian, particularly with certain racial groups, is recommended if simple measures fail.

Alcohol

Alcohol in moderation (two or three units a day) reduces cardiovascular risk, whereas excess alcohol or binge drinking increases risk. Alcohol is an important cause of weight gain and poor diabetic control which should be taken into account. Alcohol is not a medicine!

Physical activity

Regular dynamic exercise should be encouraged. Walking as briskly as possible, swimming or cycling are effective everyday forms of exercise that can help with weight control, lipids, glucose tolerance and blood pressure. Ideally 40 minutes of exercise five times a week should be aimed for. An exercise ECG can be of help in assessing the degree of exercise that can be safely undertaken (e.g. before going skiing or taking up running). If weight loss is needed, daily exercise time should increase to 60–90 minutes.

Stress

The place of stress as an independent risk factor for CAD is unclear, but there is no doubt that it provokes angina and almost certainly worsens other risk factors. The diagnosis of angina itself is stressful and although patients usually benefit from reassurance it is important that they look at their lifestyle, workload and leisure time. Controlling stress with relaxation techniques and audio tapes has been shown to be helpful.

Hypertension

Hypertension is an important cause of CAD and stroke. There is clear evidence of benefit from antihypertensive therapy (Figure 10). The drugs of choice in patients with both hypertension and angina are beta-blockers and calcium antagonists. Controlling hypertension may relieve anginal symptoms and improve physical activity. The target blood pressure is < 140/90 mmHg, with an ideal of 130/80 mmHg or less in non-diabetics. Diabetics, those with known CAD or chronic renal disease should be below 130/80 mmHg with the risk benefit continuing down to 115/75 mmHg.

Antioxidants

There is no evidence of benefit from antioxidant supplements (e.g. vitamins E, C and beta-carotene).

Diabetes

Diabetic patients are at a significantly increased risk of cardiovascular disease. Intensive glucose control reduces microvascular complications and possibly macrovascular complications. Diabetic patients (insulin-dependent or non-insulin-dependent) benefit from aggressive risk-factor control, including lipid-lowering therapy, blood pressure control and cessation of smoking.

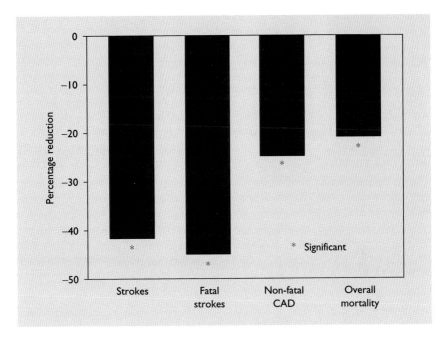

Figure 10 Benefits of treating hypertension. A meta-analysis of 14 randomized trials looked at 370 000 patients, 47% of whom were women, and concluded that when hypertension was controlled: • strokes were reduced by 42% (significant); • fatal strokes were reduced by 45% (significant); • non-fatal CAD was reduced by 14% (significant); • overall cardiovascular mortality was reduced by 21% (significant). (MacMahon et al. Blood pressure stroke and coronary heart disease. Lancet 1990; 355: 765–74.)

Hormone replacement therapy

The debate continues regarding hormone replacement therapy (HRT). It is clearly not a form of secondary prevention for CHD. In the latest publication from the Womens Health Initiative (WHI), women aged 50–59 years at entry had less calcified plaque burden when allocated oestrogen compared to placebo. This reassuring finding should allay the fears of women who need HRT for menopausal symptoms. Healthy women in the early phase of the menopause are at low absolute risk whether on HRT or not. HRT can be safely prescribed for women with menopausal symptoms using the lowest effective dose for as short an interval as possible. Low-dose vaginal oestrogen is not significantly absorbed into the systemic circulation and could therefore be continued long term for persistent and distressing vaginal symptoms.

- HRT is not recommended for primary or secondary prevention of CHD

Lipids

Hyperlipidaemia is common, with over half of men in the UK having a cholesterol level of 6.5 mmol/l or greater. Familial hypercholesterolaemia affects 2% of the population and is associated with a significantly increased risk of CAD.

A lipid-profile fasting (≥ 9 hours) is recommended for all patients with angina or with other evidence of CAD and for those at high risk of developing atheroma. It is the overall risk that is important. Screening total cholesterol and HDL cholesterol can be taken non-fasting. There is now overwhelming evidence that lipid-lowering therapy reduces the risk of major coronary events (coronary death and non-fatal myocardial infarction) by 34%, coronary mortality by 42%, the need for PCI or CABG by 37% and overall mortality by 30%.

- LDL cholesterol increases CAD risk (Figure 11)
- HDL cholesterol reduces CAD risk
- Women have higher levels of HDL before the menopause; in women a high HDL level (> 1.3 mmol/l) may protect from a rising LDL
- It is important to know a full lipid profile since different drugs have different effects on the various components

It is perhaps not fully appreciated that 80% of patients who develop CAD have a total plasma cholesterol level that is within a similar range to those who do not develop CAD. In other words, most people who develop CAD do not have very high cholesterol levels but it is too high for them as individuals.

Evidence of benefit

Statins (hydroxymethyl glutaryl coenzyme A reductase inhibitors) reduce the risk of CVD complications in both the primary and secondary setting though this division is somewhat artificial. A meta-analysis of cardiovascular outcomes trials comparing intensive versus moderate statin therapy confirmed a significant benefit for the more aggressive approach for preventing predominantly non-fatal cardiovascular events.

In diabetic patients without evidence of CVD, statin therapy provided protection from major cardiac events. In well-controlled hypertensives with no cardiac history and a total cholesterol of ≤ 6.5 mmol/l, atorvastatin compared to placebo reduced CVD events by over 30%, causing the trial to be stopped after only

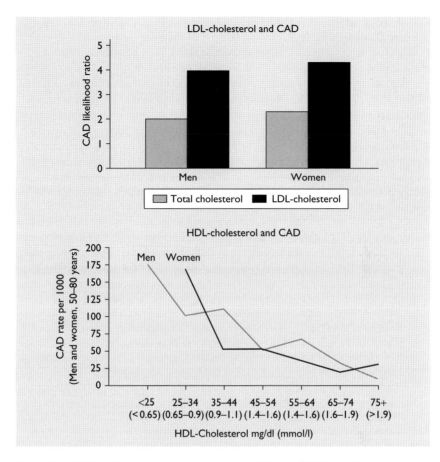

Figure 11 *(a) There is a stronger correlation between LDL and CAD than with total cholestrol. (b) HDL is a protective factor.*

3 years. There is also evidence of benefit in those up to 85 years of age who have a CAD history.

The guideline targets change as each publication adds to the evidence base, but at present they are as follows:

- *Low risk.* Lifestyle advice (weight, diet, physical activity): target total cholesterol of <5 mmol/l (190 mg/dl): LDL cholesterol <3 mmol/l (115 mg/dl): triglycerides <1.7 mmol/l (150 mg/dl) and HDL cholesterol >1 mmol/l (40 mg/dl) in men and >1.2 mmol/l (45 mg/dl) in women. Introduce statin therapy if risk after lifestyle changes for 3–6 months is over 20% (10 years CVD event rate).

- *High risk*. Established CVD, diabetes, chronic renal disease, hypertension. Lifestyle advice combined with statin therapy: target total cholesterol < 4 mmol/l (155 mg/dl) LDL cholesterol < 2 mmol/l (80 mg/dl) with an ideal LDL < 1.8 mmol/l (70 mg/dl).

The statins have beneficial actions other than lowering LDL cholesterol (reducing inflammatory markers such as C-reactive protein), and there are differences between them in terms of potency, drug interactions and blood–brain barrier penetration (with possible side-effect implications). They are safe and effective biochemically and clinically. Occasionally, a reversible elevation in liver enymes occurs usually within 6 months of initiating therapy. Myalgia and rarely myositis (creatine phosphokinase becomes elevated) may occur. The clinical benefit stems from stabilizing mild to moderately severe atheromatous plaques, so making them less vulnerable to rupture and less likely to provoke thrombosis.

Practical advice on lipids

- Check the lipids, monitor the response and, when stable and acceptable, check at 6–12-monthly intervals. Monitor liver function at each dose titration point
- Diet alone reduces cholesterol by at most 10%, so it is rarely the answer alone but it may reduce drug requirements
- Preparations containing phyto-oestrogens may assist dietary changes
- Statins are effective in 21 days and need to be titrated to targets
- Fluvastatin (40–80 mg) avoids drug interactions and is less likely to induce muscular pain
- Pravastatin (10–40 mg), simvastatin (10–40 mg) and atorvastatin (10–80 mg) are proven effective agents in large research trials
- Rosuvastatin (5–40 mg) is the most potent statin
- Statins have little impact on HDL, whereas fibrates elevate this by up to 30% and lower triglycerides by 30%. Fibrates do not reduce CVD events on their own
- Consider fibrates when HDL < 1.00 mmol/l and triglycerides > 2.00 mmol/l
- Fibrates (e.g. bezafibrate, fenofibrate or ciprofibrate) can be used in combination with statins but myalgia may occur more frequently
- Always check for secondary causes, in particular hypothyroidism, diabetes and excess alcohol intake
- Most patients will respond to simvastatin or atorvastatin
- Refer to your lipid clinic if abnormalities fail to respond or if you are unsure about management
- Although adverse effects are unusual, they should be looked for as they do vary between products. Erectile dysfunction has been reported
- Sleep and mood disturbance may occur with simvastatin and atorvastatin
- Ezetimibe 10 mg, a cholesterol sequestering agent, can be added to statins if targets have not been reached or used if statin intolerant

Advice on daily living

Driving

Patients with stable angina are allowed to drive cars but not heavy goods or public service vehicles. If angina occurs on driving, driving should be stopped. All patients should check with their personal insurers. Ambulance, fire, police, taxi and hire-car drivers with angina are also advised not to drive professionally (see Table 11, p 69).

Work

Heavy labouring jobs are likely to induce pain and may need to be changed: otherwise, stable angina does not usually influence employment, and 90% of patients can continue to work. Where employment stress is a particular problem, early retirement should be considered if a favourable financial package is available. Sympathetic employers may allow part-time work for more restricted patients. Full-time housewives may need help with heavier jobs.

Sex

Sex, like any form of exercise, can induce pain. The stress on the heart is equivalent to briskly (in 10 seconds) climbing two flights (12 steps each) of stairs. An alternative test is walking 1 mile on the level in 20 minutes. A simple test is therefore possible and if pain occurs it can be repeated with GTN beforehand. GTN can be used effectively before sexual intercourse.

The bedroom and the sheets should be warm. Sex should be avoided within 1 hour of a large meal or a hot bath. Positions within the bounds of common sense do not matter. Casual sex is more stressful. Advice is the same for heterosexuals and homosexuals.

- The chance of a cardiac event during sex between partners who have a long-standing relationship is < 1%

Sex may be avoided because of drug-induced male impotence (erectile dysfunction), which should always be asked about. Drug-induced female sexual effects definitely occur but have not been the subject of study.

Sildenafil (Viagra), tadalafil (Cialis), vardenafil (Levitra)—phosphodiesterase type 5 inhibitors

Erectile dysfunction (ED) is strongly associated with age, with estimated prevalence rates of 39% in men between 40 and 70 years of age and of 67% in those over 70 years of age. In addition to age, risk factors for ED include heart disease, hypertension, diabetes, depression and cigarette smoking, and it may be a consequence of drug therapy. Because ED and CAD share several risk factors they often coexist. Phosphodiesterase type 5 (PDE5) inhibitors increase blood flow and engorgement of the penis. Cardiovascular risks appear to be no more than placebo, providing that patients are properly advised and assessed. Nitrates act through the same biochemical pathway and the combination of nitrates and a PDE5 inhibitor can cause a critical and potentially fatal fall in blood pressure. Long-acting oral nitrates should be discontinued for 5 days before and sublingual nitrates avoided for 24 hours before and after the use of a PDE5 inhibitor.

All three PDE5 inhibitors are highly effective in restoring erectile function in up to 80% of men with CVD. The major differences are in speed and duration of action. Over 50% of men with CVD have ED and in half of these the ED begins 2–3 years before a cardiac event.

Practical points

- ED is common and causes significant distress to the man and partner
- ED may present before CVD, so that cardiac risk needs to be assessed in all cases
- PDE5 inhibitors are very effective. Sildenafil and vardenafil achieve full effect 1 hour after ingestion, with a duration of action of 6–8 hours. Tadalafil is effective after 2 hours, with a duration of action of 36–48 hours. All these drugs need stimulation to be effective
- PDE5 inhibitors may not work initially, so up to 7–8 attempts on separate days may be needed
- Side effects include flushing, headache, nasal congestion and acid reflux, but PDE5 inhibitors are usually well tolerated. Back pain can occur with tadalafil
- If these drugs are not successful, other options include vacuum pumps, constriction rings and cavernosal injection therapy
- If libido is reduced check testosterone (before 10 am)
- Female sexual dysfunction (FSD) is also common but is more complex to treat. Specialist referral is advised
- PDE5 inhibitors are effective, well-tolerated and safe therapies for men with ED for the general population, including those with CAD, providing that they are thoroughly assessed
- The use of any form of nitrates and nicorandil is an absolute contraindication
- Stable angina patients not taking nitrates and with a good exercise ability are not at increased risk—use the stair test or walking test
- If in doubt about safety, refer for an exercise test—sex is the equivalent to 3–4 minutes on the treadmill (Bruce protocol)—or a formal cardiological opinion. Doing the exercise test in the presence of a partner may reduce the partner's anxiety also

Key points

- Prevention is fundamental
- Lipid control is essential
- No risk factor should be judged in isolation—a multifactorial disease needs comprehensive action
- The cholesterol at which CAD developed was too high for that individual – it's not just the number, it's the person.
- The detection, management and education about risk factors and CAD prevention represents a very important role for the GP and the practice team
- Stable angina should not restrict a normal life which includes a normal sex and working life

Drug therapy

Drugs can be used for symptom relief, prognosis or both. Grapefruit juice can influence the metabolism of many drugs and patients should be asked to avoid it. Lipid lowering has been covered on pages 40–42. A regular audit of drug therapy is recommended—e.g. What percentage of patients are on aspirin? What percentage have achieved their lipid-lowering target?

Aspirin

A review of the trials of aspirin in patients with stable angina showed a reduction in the risk of vascular death, stroke and myocardial infarction of 25%. An initial dose of 300 mg maximizes the inhibition of platelet aggregation, and 75 mg daily then maintains it.

Absolute contraindications are few and include active peptic ulceration (enteric coating is of no significant benefit), aspirin hypersensitivity and aspirin-induced asthma.

- Treating 1000 patients at high risk for 2 years will prevent 40 vascular deaths
- There is no convincing evidence that a 75 mg dosage of enteric-coated agents reduces the risk of major gastrointestinal bleeding
- Alka-Seltzer is an alternative means of taking aspirin and is preferred by some patients
- Aspirin should be routinely recommended
- Intracranial bleeding is less than 1 per 1000 patient-years at 75 mg dosage
- In patients with gastroduodenal ulcers, esomeprazole 40 mg (a proton pump inhibitor) is effective in preventing recurrent ulcer bleeding

Clopidogrel, 75 mg daily, is an alternative agent for those who are intolerant of or unsuitable for aspirin. Dipyridamole is not recommended due to uncertain efficacy and potentially causing coronary steal.

ACE Inhibitors

Whilst there is no doubt ACE inhibitors are of benefit in the presences of reduced left ventricular systolic function, their use in the presence of good left ventricular function remains controversial. However, meta-analyses have shown ACE

Antiplatelets Trialists Collaboration. Secondary prevention of vascular disease by prolonged antiplatelet treatment. BMJ 1988; 296: 320–31.

Table 7 Nitrate preparations

Preparation	Use	Comments
Sublingual GTN tablets 500 µg	Alleviates attacks quickly. Prophylaxis 30 minutes	Causes headaches. Replenish every 2 months. Careful storage needed
GTN spray 400 µg	Alleviates attacks quickly. Prophylaxis 30 minutes	Convenient Expensive. Causes headaches. Inflammable
Topical nitrates	Nocturnal symptoms? Debatable whether they are useful	Expensive. Intermittent use to avoid tolerance Patch is cosmetically better than paste
Isosorbide dinitrate (sublingual or oral)	Sublingual prophylaxis 1 hour. Oral prevention of pain. 10–40 mg bd or long-acting formulations	As GTN. Hepatic metabolism leads to varying effectiveness
Isosorbide mononitrate (oral)	Prevention of pain 10–40 mg bd or long acting formulations	100% bioavailability. Preferable to dinitrate
Buccal nitrates	Alleviates pain. Prophylaxis	Expensive. Variably tolerated. Useful when oral therapy is not possible

inhibitors significantly reduce cardiovascular and all-cause mortality, non-fatal myocardial infarction and stroke when the left ventricular systolic function is well-preserved. ACE inhibitors should be routinely prescribed in patients with angina and co-existing ventricular dysfunction, hypertension or diabetes and considered for all patients with stable angina. In stable angina patients without co-existing indications for ACE-inhibitors however their use should be set against side-effects, cost and adherence to therapy.

Antianginal drugs

Every patient is an individual and responses will vary; however, there remains a reluctance on the one hand to use drugs optimally, reflected most often in the underdosing of beta-blockers, and on the other hand a random adding on of therapy without stopping ineffective agents, leading to so-called triple therapy. An overview is provided in Figure 12.

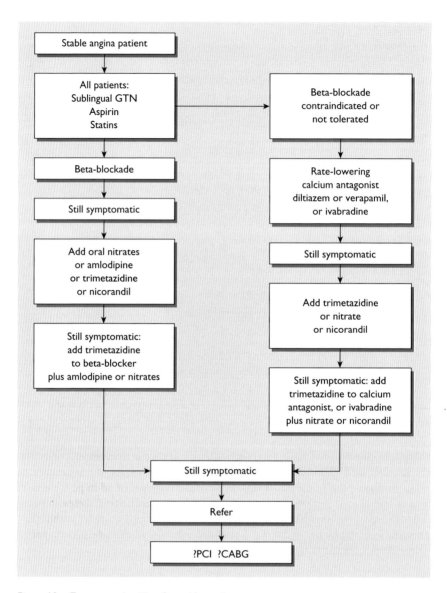

Figure 12 Treatment algorithm for stable angina.

Nitrates

Nitrates are vascular smooth muscle relaxants (Table 7). They act mainly on veins and to a lesser extent on arteries and they are of benefit in angina because they cause peripheral vasodilatation, which reduces myocardial work and thereby oxygen demand, and coronary dilatation, which improves myocardial blood flow. Nitrates are also inhibitors of platelet aggregation, which may be important in unstable angina.

Sublingual nitrates

Sublingual nitrates avoid hepatic metabolism. All patients should be prescribed and instructed in the use of sublingual nitrates either to relieve pain or as prophylaxis. They work rapidly (in 1–2 minutes) with a 30-minute duration of effect.

The GTN spray is more expensive but has a longer storage life (2 years) than the GTN tablets (8 weeks).

GTN tablets must be stored in an airtight bottle without cotton wool and kept in a cool place. An active tablet has a burning effect on the tongue—tell the patient to get a fresh supply if this is not experienced.

- A GTN spray should be in a GP's emergency bag

Buccal nitrates

A sustained-release formulation of GTN is available. This is placed between the upper lip and the gum. The dosage is 1 mg, 2 mg, 3 mg or 5 mg. It lasts up to 4 hours and can be of value in unstable angina and heart failure. Tolerance is not usually a problem. Pre- and postoperative use when patients are 'nil by mouth' and nocturnal use in severe cases are other indications. This formulation is expensive and not popular with patients.

Long-acting nitrates

Oral 5-isosorbide mononitrate (5-ISMN) gives more consistent blood levels than the dinitrate, which relies on hepatic metabolism for conversion to the active mononitrate. Nitrate tolerance (decreasing effect with time) is avoided by asymmetric (8.00 am and 2.00 pm) or 12-hourly dosing or once-daily slow-release preparations, which have a low nitrate trough point.

Doses advised are:

- conventional mononitrate 10 mg, 20 mg (usually optimal) or 40 mg bd
- once-daily preparations: 25 mg, 40 mg, 50 mg or 60 mg 5-ISMN

Tolerance can be successfully overcome by using daily dosing regimens that include a nitrate-low interval—a period of 8–12 hours each day during which plasma nitrate levels are sufficiently low to prevent the development of tolerance.

Patient compliance is a key factor in the successful management of angina. Patients with angina often receive concomitant therapy for their symptoms and therefore benefit from simple dosing regimens. Therefore, to encourage good patient compliance and to maximize the benefits of angina prophylaxis, the most practical and convenient solution is to administer the nitrate in a simple once-daily formulation. Nitrates can be safely used in combination with beta-blockers, calcium antagonists and trimetazidine (page 59) and when there is significant left ventricular dysfunction or cardiac failure.

- Conventional mononitrate can be titrated from 10 mg bd to 20 and then 40 mg bd
- Allow 12 hours between doses or use asymmetrical dosing, e.g. 8 am and 2 pm
- Most benefit is at 20 mg bd
- Once-daily preparations are a convenient alternative as 25 mg, 40 mg, 50 mg or 60 mg preparations—reducing tolerance and increasing compliance

Topical nitrates

Topical nitrates avoid hepatic metabolism, but consistent blood levels lead to rapid tolerance. Intermittent use (12 hours on, 12 hours off) is effective but expensive. Dosage is 5 mg, 10 mg or 15 mg.

- Because topical nitrates require nitrate-free periods to be effective they cannot be used safely as monotherapy

They may help nocturnal pain (when put on at night, and taken off in the morning). The location of the patch is not important, but there is psychological benefit if it is put on the chest.

Side effects

About 10% of patients cannot take nitrates because of side effects. The commonest is headache, which the patient should be warned about. Syncope rarely occurs and is more common in the elderly and after alcohol. Other side effects include flushing and halitosis with sublingual tablets. Nitrates are contraindicated in hypertrophic obstructive cardiomyopathy—a rare cause of angina. Nitrates are contraindicated when a PDE5 inhibitor is prescribed and vice versa.

Beta-blockers

Beta-blockers (Table 8) are very important antianginal drugs because of their cardioprotective properties:

Table 8 Features of beta-blockers indicated for stable angina

Drug	Potency	Cardio-selective	Optimum dose pharmaco-dynamic half-life (hours)	Blood–brain barrier penetration	Dosage adjustment
Acebutolol	0.3*	+	24	NS	In renal impairment
Atenolol	1	+	24	NS	In renal impairment
Bisoprolol	10	+	24	Yes	—
Metoprolol	1	+	10–12	Yes	In hepatic impairment
Nadolol	1.5	–	39	NS	In renal impairment
Oxprenolol	0.5–1.0*	–	13	Yes	In hepatic impairment
Pindolol	6*	–	8	Yes	—
Propranolol	1	–	11	Yes	In hepatic impairment
Timolol	6	–	15	Yes	In hepatic impairment

NS: not significant.
*Agents with partial agonist activity.

- after myocardial infarction, they improve prognosis
- they are antiarrhythmic and reduce the risk of ventricular fibrillation
- they reduce the risk of reinfarction
- they improve prognosis in compensated cardiac failure
- they do not improve prognosis in stable angina with a normal left ventricle.

Beta-blockers are effective in more than 90% of angina patients and should be considered for prescription immediately the diagnosis has been made. They are effective in all age groups, in both sexes, and in smokers and non-smokers.

Beta-blockers benefit ischaemia by prolonging coronary filling as a result of slowing the heart rate and reducing myocardial demand by lowering blood pressure and myocardial contractility. They reduce the anginal attack rate and GTN consumption as well as increasing exercise ability. Exercise ECGs show less ST depression and 24-hour ECGs show fewer episodes of painful or silent ischaemia. The single most important reason for ineffectiveness is inadequate dosage. The patient's resting heart rate is a simple measure of beta-blockade, but the exercise heart rate is a better guide.

- A resting heart rate of 50 beats per minute is not an indication for dosage reduction unless there are symptoms of lethargy or excessive fatigue

Propranolol is the reference drug, with a potency of 1. It can be given twice daily (half-life 11 hours). Atenolol is equal in potency but with a half-life of 24 hours can be given once daily.

Cardioselectivity

This is relative and indicates a preference for beta-1-receptors in the heart versus beta-2-receptors in the lungs or periphery. As the dose of a selective agent increases, the degree of selectivity decreases. The reduced effect on the beta-2-peripheral vessels can be helpful in promoting better hypotensive effects (e.g. atenolol, metoprolol), but postural changes are less likely with non-selective agents (peripheral vasoconstriction).

Lipophilicity

Lipid-soluble agents pass through the liver and enter the brain more than water-soluble (hydrophilic) agents. This can lead to adverse effects (e.g. dreams, concentration difficulties) but may be an advantage if anxiety is a particular problem (propanolol is useful in this regard).

Partial agonist activity

Also known as intrinsic sympathomimetic activity (ISA), partial agonist activity (PAA) is a partial stimulant effect that leads to less detrimental effect on cardiac

Table 9 *Adverse effects of beta-blockers*

- Most side effects are predictable from our knowledge of the sympathetic nervous system
- They are contraindicated in the presence of second- or third-degree heart block, but not in first-degree or left bundle branch block
- They may induce bronchospasm, less so if selective, and are contraindicated in asthma
- Fatigue, depression or a 'zombie-like' feeling are fairly common
- Cold hands and feet and heavy legs reflect a fall in cardiac output and can be helped by co-prescribing with a vasodilator
- Hydrophilic agents are likely to accumulate in renal dysfunction and lipophilic agents are likely to accumulate in hepatic dysfunction
- ED, which may be related to the reduction in cardiac output, affects 10% of patients and should be routinely asked about. Beta-blockers are prognostically important for many patients. So if ED occurs a PDE5 inhibitor should be prescribed and the beta-blocker continued
- There are small adverse effects on cholesterol and HDL cholesterol and, more significantly, on triglycerides. These are theoretically important, but they do not outweigh the proven advantages. They are corrected by statins
- Diabetic persons who are prone to hypoglycaemia may have their warning symptoms masked, except for perspiration. Non-selective agents prolong hypoglycaemia in patients receiving insulin and reduce the tachycardia. These effects are less with a cardioselective agent. Beta-blockers do not increase the frequency of hypoglycaemic episodes but may worsen glucose intolerance. Diabetic persons can be prescribed cardioselective beta-blockers, but care is needed when the diabetes is insulin-dependent

Note that beta-blockers should not be stopped abruptly because a rebound effect may occur, leading to unstable angina or infarction.

output and the periphery. There is increasing PAA with dosage increase, so the level of beta-blockade usually reaches a plateau at 80% of maximum. Agents with PAA (e.g. acebutolol) cause less bradycardia and cold peripheries, but those with more PAA have less hypotensive properties.

Adverse effects

The adverse effects are largely predictable and often caused by inappropriate patient selection (Table 9). It is not logical to use even cardioselective beta-blockers in a patient with bronchospasm without using nitrates and calcium antagonists as a safer initial option.

Using beta-blockers

The following points represent my personal preferences. Use agents that are cardio-selective and preferably hydrophilic, once or twice daily. Stick to one or two drugs and use them optimally.

Atenolol is cardioselective and hydrophilic, and it works once daily at 50 mg, 100 mg and 200 mg but twice daily at 25 mg dosage. Peak blood levels occur 3–4 hours after the dose and correlate with fatigue side effects. Therefore it is often prescribed in the evening. Begin at 25 mg in the elderly and 50 mg in those aged below 70 years.

Propranolol is highly lipophilic and should be used principally when there is a high level of anxiety or postural hypotension. The dose is 40, 80 or 160 mg bd. Once-daily long-acting formulations aid adherence to therapy (80 and 160 mg LA). Bisoprolol is a convenient once-daily cardioselective beta-blocker with low-dose flexibility reducing adverse effects especially in the elderly (doses are 1.25, 2.5, 5 and 10 mg daily).

Acebutolol is cardioselective and hydrophilic with PAA. It is a twice- or once-daily agent, depending on dose. Use it when peripheral adverse effects are a problem or likely to be so (e.g. with coexisting claudication). It is not as effective in severe cases since the resting heart rate is not suppressed to the same degree. The dose is 100 mg bd, 200 mg bd and 400 mg once or twice daily.

Beta-blockers are first-line agents for stable angina.

- All patients with stable angina should be considered for beta-blockade at the same time as sublingual nitrates are prescribed
- Beta-blockers should not be stopped abruptly since a rebound effect may occur, leading to unstable angina or infarction
- Calcium antagonists do not protect from rebound
- Beta-blockers in low dosage are used in controlled heart failure to improve prognosis

Beta-blockers should not be suddenly withdrawn because rebound effects can occur, leading to unstable angina or myocardial infarction. This is less of a problem with long-acting agents such as atenolol or less potent agents with PAA.

Beta-blockers all share the same mechanism of action—competition at the beta-receptor—so full effect depends on optimal dosage.

Labetalol and Carvedilol are combined beta- and alpha-blockers and also approved for treating angina but are best reserved for patients in whom hypertension and angina coexist.

Calcium antagonists

Since they were first introduced in the 1960s, these drugs have proven to be effective in the management of chronic stable angina and hypertension. They do not protect the patient from abrupt withdrawal of beta-blockade.

Safety

Anxieties about the calcium antagonists relate to the short-acting dihydropyridines, which are not advocated for angina as monotherapy because their rapid onset of action induces a reflex tachycardia, which may bring on anginal pain. Longer-acting agents present no increased risk, nor do the heart rate-lowering agents diltiazem and verapamil.

Actions

Calcium ions are essential for myocardial contraction and conduction. Calcium antagonists act by impairing the influx of these ions into smooth muscle, myocardial cells and conducting tissue cells. The effects can be summarized: myocardial contractility may be reduced; conduction may be depressed; and coronary and peripheral vascular tone is relaxed.

Different calcium antagonists have different properties and these variations are extremely important—much more important than the differences between beta-blockers (Table 10).

Diltiazem and verapamil reduce heart rate, atrioventricular conduction and cardiac output. Diltiazem has more effect on the sinoatrial node than verapamil but less effect on atrioventricular conduction and cardiac output. Both have modest peripheral dilating effects, diltiazem more than verapamil.

The dihydropyridine calcium-channel antagonists (amlodipine, felodipine, isradipine, lacidipine, nicardipine, nifedipine and nisoldipine) are principally peripheral and coronary vasodilators. They are less likely to depress cardiac output because any deleterious effects are offset by afterload reduction resulting from peripheral vasodilatation. Caution is strongly advised in the presence of significant left ventricular dysfunction, however, particularly if combined with beta-blockade. They have no effect on cardiac conduction. The agents that are

Table 10 Properties of calcium antagonists. Diltiazem lowers resting heart rate proportionally. The higher the resting heart rate, the more it is lowered

Effect on	Nisoldipine, felodipine, amlodipine	Nifedipine, nicardipine	Long-acting nifedipine	Verapamil	Diltiazem
Heart rate	0 (⇑)	⇑⇑	0 (⇑)	0 ⇩	0 ⇩
Atrioventricular conduction	0	0	0	⇩⇩	⇨
Peripheral vasodilation	+++	+++	+++	++	++
Coronary vasodilation	+++	+++	+++	++	+++
Contractility	0 (⇩)	(⇩) 0	(⇩) 0	⇩⇩	⇨

currently approved for angina are amlodipine, felodipine, nifedipine, nisoldipine and nicardipine.

Using calcium antagonists

Calcium antagonists have gained widespread acceptance for the treatment of angina because of their proven efficacy and their lack of the fatiguing side effects that unfortunately limit beta-blockade. In addition, their vasodilating properties may be beneficial in Raynaud's phenomenon and when bronchospasm is a problem. Diltiazem and verapamil may be used in non-Q-wave infarction for prevention of reinfarction, providing that left ventricular function is good. Diltiazem has been reported as reducing reinfarction and improving cardiac function after myocardial infarction.

In general, calcium antagonists can be advocated:

- as an alternative to beta-blockade, particularly a heart rate-lowering calcium-channel blocker (diltiazem, verapamil)
- when beta-blockers are contraindicated
- when beta-blockers induce adverse effects
- in addition to nitrates and trimetazidine
- in addition to beta-blockers, though only dihydropyridines are totally safe because a conduction interaction is absent. Verapamil should be avoided and diltiazem should be used very carefully
- when bronchospasm is also present because of potentially beneficial actions on bronchial smooth muscle tone as well as angina

Verapamil is a powerful antiarrhythmic drug that is particularly suitable for supraventricular tachycardias. It has comparable efficacy to beta-blockers as monotherapy, but it is not safe to co-prescribe with a beta-blocker. It is the most cardiac depressant of the calcium antagonists. There is a significant interaction with digoxin, which may affect atrioventricular conduction and increase digoxin levels and side effects. Slow-release formulations are available: 120–480 mg daily.

Adverse effects of verapamil include flushing and headaches secondary to vasodilatation and constipation (especially in the elderly). High-fibre diets may help, but constipation can be severe and verapamil must be discontinued in these cases. Verapamil rarely impairs liver function. Although it causes fluid retention and vasodilatation side effects, these are less than with dihydropyridines.

Diltiazem is similar to verapamil but causes less depression of atrioventricular conduction and cardiac contraction. It is an effective monotherapy in angina, equivalent to beta-blockade. In patients with chronic stable angina, it reduces resting heart rate, particularly in those with a high heart rate at baseline, but it does not prevent the increase in heart rate in response to exercise. It has also been shown to reduce the frequency of anginal attacks and nitrate consumption and increase exercise time in such patients.

The adverse effects of diltiazem are less than those of verapamil, with less constipation reported.

Once-daily formulations of diltiazem have proven and published independent data supporting their 24-hour cover and may be preferred.

Dihydropyridines for angina pectoris include amlodipine, felodipine, nicardipine, nisoldipine and nifedipine. They are potent arterial vasodilators that act by relaxing vascular smooth muscle. There is less effect on myocardial contraction but their use is still unwise if left ventricular function is substantially impaired. They have no antiarrhythmic actions and are safe with beta-blockade. They are especially effective when coronary spasm is considered a component. However, this is rare (<5% of cases) in stable angina.

Their adverse effects reflect more vasodilatation; therefore it is more likely for there to be flushing, headaches and diuretic-resistant fluid retention (at the ankles and/or abdomen). Eye pain and gum hyperplasia are reported with nifedipine and amlodipine. Occasionally, ischaemic pain can follow the ingestion of short-acting preparations of nifedipine and nicardipine. This may reflect the drugs' rapid onset of action involving a heart rate increase or a coronary steal effect. Long-acting preparations are preferred for this reason.

No lipid adverse effects have been reported with calcium antagonists. The drugs are not as effective as beta-blockers in smokers.

Sorting out the differences

Diltiazem and verapamil should mainly be seen as alternatives to beta-blockers.

The currently approved dihydropyridines are very similar in action. Little difference exists between the long-acting preparations, all of which are equally as effective as nitrates as monotherapy but less effective than beta-blockade.

Dosage guidelines

When using calcium antagonists the following guidelines are suggested.

- Verapamil and diltiazem should mainly be seen as effective alternatives to beta-blockers. Verapamil should not be co-prescribed with a beta-blocker because of an unpredictable interaction on conduction. The verapamil dose is 40–160 mg tds or, for slow-release preparations, 120 mg or 240 mg bd

- Diltiazem may be used cautiously with beta-blockers. There are various retard preparations (90 mg or 120 mg bd) and long-acting formulations (LA 200 mg or LA 300 mg). It is well tolerated in all age groups
- Nifedipine is convenient in the retard preparation (10 mg or 20 mg bd, in the elderly begin with 10 mg bd)
- Nicardipine is inconvenient. The dose is 20 mg tds, increasing to 40 mg tds. No significant advantage in its formulation justifies its use above nifedipine or amlodipine
- Shorter-acting agents (nifedipine, nicardipine and isradipine) can induce angina as a result of reflex tachycardia. They should not be used as monotherapy but are safe in combination with beta-blockade
- Longer-acting dihydropyridines are safer than short-acting agents and avoid the tendency to reflex tachycardia (and thereby chest pain) in the absence of beta-blockers. They are effective in combination with beta-blockers. Examples are amlodipine 5–10 mg, nifedipine LA 30–60 mg, felodipine 5–20 mg once daily and nisoldipine 10–40 mg once daily
- Care should be taken when angina and heart failure coexist. Amlodipine and felodipine do not worsen or improve heart failure survival but they can be used if pain is a complication when the failure is controlled. Be on the alert for an additive hypotensive effect with ACE inhibitors

Key points

- Calcium antagonists are important alternatives to beta-blockers
- Avoid short-acting agents

Nicorandil

This is a potassium-channel activator with actions similar to both nitrates and calcium antagonists. It is equal in effectiveness to beta-blockers, calcium antagonists or nitrates, with headache (usually short-lived but occasionally severe) as its commonest side effect. Reflex tachycardia is not reported and no metabolic problems have been documented. It does not depress left ventricular function or cause peripheral oedema. Tolerance occasionally occurs.

The dose is 10–30 mg bd. It is an alternative agent when others are contraindicated or cause side effects and it can be used in combination with nitrates, beta-blockers and calcium antagonists. Its present role is not first line because of the absence of convincing prognostic data, and although it is as effective as other agents, it is not more effective. PDE5 inhibitors are contraindicated in the presence of nicroandil.

Metabolic agents

These act at a cellular level, reducing ischaemia by increasing glucose metabolism relative to free fatty acids, and thereby increasing adenosine triphosphate generation per unit of oxygen consumption.

Trimetazidine

Trimetazidine (20 mg tds or 35 mg MR bd) has antianginal efficacy equivalent to oral nitrates, calcium antagonists and beta-blockers. It has no haemodynamic effects, and it is very effective in combination with haemodynamic agents such as the beta-blockers, calcium antagonists and nitrates. It is safe and effective in the presence of cardiac failure and has been shown to improve ejection fraction. In two small studies prognosis was also improved. It does not react with PDE5 inhibitors so can replace nitrates or nicorandil to allow for their safe use in treating ED. Side effects are minimal (equivalent to placebo) and it is very well tolerated in the elderly.

- Trimetazidine can be used as add-on therapy to conventional haemodynamic agents or used as monotherapy when they are not tolerated (Figure 12)
- Trimetazidine is safe in the presence of cardiac failure and improves ejection fraction as well as symptoms
- In a Cochrane meta-analysis of 23 studies involving 1378 patients, trimetazidine significantly reduced angina attacks, and increased exercise time to 1 mm ST depression when compared with placebo. Side effects were no more than placebo

Ranolozine

Originally thought to act like trimetazidine, ranolozine is now believed to inhibit the late sodium current (I_{Na}) and the accumulation of intracellular sodium and calcium overload. Ischaemia-induced decreased compliance increased LV stiffness and capillary compression is reversed without any reduction in systolic function (in contrast to beta-blockers and calcium antagonists).

Clinical studies have demonstrated symptomatic antianginal benefit and improved exercise tolerance as monotherapy or in combination with haemodynamic agents. No mortality data are available but a consistent lowering of haemoglobin A_{IC} in diabetics has been observed. Adverse effects include constipation, nausea and dizziness (syncope has been recorded). Ranolozine increases the QT interval and, though torsades de pointes has not been recorded, caution is advised in patients taking other drugs that may prolong the QT interval or influence its metabolism (via CYP3A) such as diltiazem. Currently it is only available in the United States.

Ivabradine

Ivabradine is a sinus node inhibitor. It selectively and specifically inhibits the I_f pacemaker current of sinoatrial cells. It produces dose-dependent (5–7.5 mg bd) improvements in exercise ability and time to ischaemia. It does not lower blood pressure. The antianginal and antiischaemic benefits of ivabradine have been evaluated in randomized controlled trials versus calcium antagonists and beta-blockers. The prognostic benefits of ivabradine are currently being evaluated. It is well tolerated with transient visual symptoms being the most frequent adverse effect. However, these symptoms do not normally lead to treatment discontinuation. Ivabradine is not recommended if atrial fibrillation is present.

Combination therapy

There is evidence of an additive effect when beta-blockers are combined with oral nitrates or calcium antagonists (not verapamil). Similarly, combining calcium antagonists with nitrates may produce an additive effect. Data on nicorandil in combination are sparse but encouraging.

There is no evidence that triple therapy or quadruple therapy is more effective than double therapy or even optimal beta-blockade as monotherapy. The idea that maximal medical therapy with as many drugs as possible is the same as optimal medical therapy is not supported by any trial data.

Beta blockers, calcium antagonists, nitrates and nicorandil all act haemodynamically prinicipally reducing oxygen demand. Once this approach is optimised adding agents with similar modes of action will confer no additional treatment and may be counterproductive introducing adverse effect.

It may be better to switch therapy within a one- or two-drug regimen rather than to continue to add various third or fourth agents.

Practical examples are:

- atenolol 50 mg or 100 mg plus amlodipine 5 mg or 10 mg per day
- atenolol 50 mg or 100 mg plus ISMN slow release 40 mg, 50 mg or 60 mg per day
- atenolol plus ISMN plus amlodipine (often used, but with no evidence to support it)

When beta-blockers are contraindicated the frequent combinations are:

- diltiazem LA 200 mg or 300 mg plus ISMN
- verapamil SR 120–240 mg bd plus ISMN
- amlodipine 5–10 mg once daily plus ISMN
- nicorandil (10–30 mg bid) may be used instead of amlodipine or ISMN
- ivabradine 5–7.5 mg bd plus amlodipine or ISMN

Atenolol plus diltiazem may be effective but runs the risk of conduction and cardiac contraction problems, particularly bradycardia. It is best initiated at atenolol 50 mg every morning and Tildiem LA 200 mg once daily to limit the potential for an adverse interaction, and dose adjustments can be made subsequently depending on effect.

- Some patients may become worse when a third agent is added to double therapy
- Always use drugs in optimal dosage but consider a combination of two low-dose drugs if side effects occur (e.g. atenolol 50 mg plus amlodipine 5 mg rather than atenolol 100 mg alone)

Using up to two haemodynamic agents may improve symptoms but a more rational approach to adding a second or third agent is to add trimetazidine which has no haemodynamic action.

- Trimetazidine added to haemodynamic agents used as monotherapy or double therapy increases exercise time, decreases exercise induced ischaemia and reduces angina attacks
- Trimetazidine is a logical additional drug when the heamodynamic options have been optimised

Simple guidelines for management

- If angina occurs in a patient with a history of a previous infarction, beta-blockers are the drugs of first choice
- Calcium antagonists, ivabradine nitrates or nicorandil can be used when beta-blockers are contraindicated (e.g. in asthma) or if they induce adverse effects (e.g. lethargy or cold peripheries)
- Combination therapy of two drugs may be additive, but triple therapy (nitrates, calcium antagonists and beta-blockers) provides little further benefit and may actually worsen the situation. Quadruple therapy with nicorandil has no data to support its use
- If there is associated heart failure, nitrates are the safest symptomatic initial anti anginal option, with low-dose beta-blockade added because of its prognostic benefit providing that the failure is controlled and the patient is stable
- Trimetazidine is effective in combination with beta blockers, nitrates, calcium antagonists and nicorandil
- Trimetazidine improves ejection fraction and has an important role in the presence of cardiac failure
- Trimetazidine is not contraindicated with a PDE5 inhibitor and can be used as a substitute for nitrates or nicorandil to allow PDE5 inhibitors to be safely prescribed.
- Ivabradine is a therapeutic alternative to beta blockers to be used in combination with nitrates, dihydropyridine calcium antagonists and trimetazidine
- When symptoms persist in spite of medical treatment, refer the patient for a cardiological opinion
- Angina needing triple therapy also needs further evaluation

Intervention

With the progress in medical therapy and the optimal evidence-based use of drug therapy, the referral for invasive revascularization has decreased. As stable patients are by definition stable, there is time to optimize care and evaluate the patients thoroughly.

Coronary artery bypass surgery (CABG) and percutaneous coronary intervention (PCI) are both effective options for the relief of anginal symptoms which should be troublesome and persistent in spite of medical therapy.

Percutaneous coronary intervention

PCI includes balloon dilatation of the coronary stenosis (often referred to as plain old balloon angioplasty—POBA) and insertion of a stent. Stents may be bare metal or drug coated—drug-eluting stents (DES). DES reduce the incidence of in-stent restenosis, which is more of a problem in longer stents (>3 cm) of small diameter (<3 mm). Reported decrease in the need for re-intervention 6–9 months after the initial procedure are from 7.1% to 10.3% for DES and from 13.3% to 18.9% for bare metal stents. Of some concern is a late thrombosis rate after DES if clopidogrel is discontinued, which is problematic if a general surgical procedure is necessary. At the present time, after DES insertion, clopidogrel and aspirin are prescribed for at least 1 year in combination and aspirin indefinitely.

PCI has given the physician, for the first time, the possibility of increasing the supply of blood to the heart rather than reducing demand. The procedure is similar to coronary angiography: the stenosis is identified, a guide wire is passed over it and a balloon is advanced along the guide wire until it crosses the lesion. The balloon is then inflated with the aim of substantially reducing the stenosis and a stent can be inserted if needed (over 90% of cases).

The primary indication for PCI is the relief of pain that has not responded to optimal medical therapy. There is a lot of information on its effectiveness, success rate and complication rate.

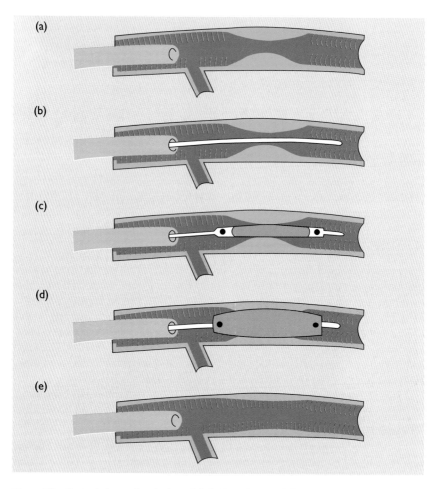

Figure 13   *The technique of angioplasty. (a) Guide catheter in left coronary artery.*
(b) Guide wire advanced through narrowing. (c) Balloon positioned with markers. (d) Balloon
inflated. (e) Catheter, with guide wire and balloon removed, leaving expanded artery.

Procedural complications have been reduced following the introduction of stents, and current figures are:

- procedural success rate: 95%
- mortality rate: <1%

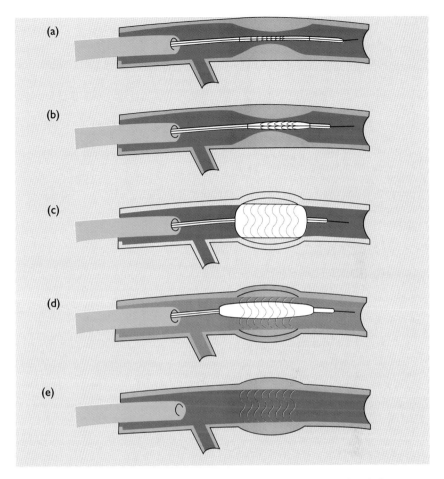

Figure 14 *The technique of stent insertion. (a) The stent (like a metal cage) on balloon catheter is positioned at the problem site. (b) The balloon catheter is then inflated. (c) The stent is fully expanded and (d) left in place after the balloon has been deflated. (e) The stent remains expanded inside the artery.*

- rate of emergency CABG: <1%
- myocardial infarct rate: <1%

The role of POBA (Figure 13) and stent placement (Figure 14) depends on how it compares with optimal medical therapy and CABG.

PCI versus medical therapy

- For patients with stable angina, there is no evidence that PCI is superior to optimal medical therapy with regard to risk of subsequent myocardial infarction or death
- PCI initially provides better relief than medical therapy from angina but after 5 years follow-up there is no difference
- PCI is principally indicated for pain relief in spite of optimal medical therapy—it is a symptom–driven alternative
- In particular, modest single-vessel disease can be safely managed medically with PCI only if symptoms persist
- There is no evidence that routine coronary stenting is superior to balloon angioplasty in terms of death, MI or the need for CABG but stents reduce the need for repeat PCI
- In-stent restenosis remains a problem reduced but not solved by DES

PCI versus CABG

- In stable patients major complications such as death and infarction are similar in frequency for PCI and CABG
- CABG involves a longer hospital stay but subsequently less angina and less antianginal drugs
- PCI is less traumatic, with only a one-night hospital stay and a rapid recovery to normal activity (day cases are increasing)
- PCI patients need more reinterventions as a result of restenosis
- PCI does not improve or worsen prognosis

Indications for PCI

- Failure of optimal medical therapy
- Suitable lesions in single or selected multivessel disease
- Angina after CABG—appropriate lesions
- Debatable—evidence of severe ischaemia on an exercise ECG in the presence of controlled symptoms medically. No evidence for this but it is often practiced

Restenosis

This continues to be a problem. It usually presents with a recurrence of angina (80%) but it can be silent. Exercise tests are not accurate in its detection. No oral drugs have reduced the incidence. PCI can be repeated five or six times with similar success and restenosis rates. Coronary stenting reduces the restenosis rate by producing larger lumens and reducing pathological remodelling.

Stents

Stents are metal cages that are expanded by a balloon to compress the stenosis. They are used to prevent acute vessel closure following PCI when a dissection has occurred and to reduce the risk of restenosis. Since they are made differently, the results for one type of stent are not necessarily applicable to others.

Stents have reduced the need for CABG when PCI is complicated by vessel closure. Stents have been shown to be more effective than PCI when treating lesions in venous bypass grafts. Though stents reduce restenosis, they do not abolish it, and restenosis within a stent can be difficult to manage. Drug-eluting stents (DES) have reduced the restenosis rate to 5–10% compared with bare-metal stents (15%), though a late thrombosis rate after clopidogrel has been stopped has caused concern. Long-term clopidogrel and aspirin are advocated but can present bleeding problems if non-cardiac surgery is contemplated. At present there is a move back from DES to bare-metal stents, especially in large diameter vessels. Primary elective stenting or direct stenting (without prior balloon dilatation) appears to reduce the complication rate of PCI and is now widely practised. The bigger the stent diameter (> 3.0 mm) and the shorter the stent (< 18 mm), the less is the chance of restenosis. Stents of ≤ 2.5 mm have an increased restenosis rate.

The major immediate limitation of coronary stenting is subacute thrombosis. This risk has been reduced through pre-treatment with clopidogrel, an antiplatelet agent, and it now averages 1%.

Clopidogrel (75 mg once daily) is prescribed with aspirin. A sensitivity reaction occasionally occurs with a florid drug rush.

Key points

- PCI relieves angina with a high initial success rate and a low complication rate
- In the absence of prognostically important disease, PCI should be advocated when symptoms persist in spite of optimal medical therapy
- Stents reduce the acute closure rate and restenosis rate
- Direct stenting reduces short-term complications and appears to have a better long-term outcome
- A combined strategy of medical therapy, risk factor modification and selective intervention based on symptoms should maximize the benefits of PCI
- The referring doctor must know the audited success rate of the local cardiovascular centres and make appropriate decisions for the individual patient
- If angina recurs after PCI the patient should be referred back
- Single-vessel disease other than in the left main stem or proximal left anterior descending artery has an excellent prognosis, so PCI with or without a stent should not be undertaken just because a lesion looks suitable

Other techniques and devices

Atherectomy, which is a technique for removing atheroma, has not been shown to offer any improvement over PCI results; it is associated with a similar restenosis rate but with more complications, and a disturbing increase in late deaths has been reported.

Lasers have demonstrated no advantages, and the rotational device for opening tough lesions has a high complication and restenosis rate.

Atherectomy and rotational devices are likely to have better defined but limited uses in the future involving DES.

Coronary surgery

The role of CABG in stable angina to relieve symptoms and to lengthen life is well established. It is effective in all age groups; those who are over 70 years of age and who are otherwise fit benefit as well as younger patients.

CABG improves survival in certain high-risk groups. CABG will relieve symptoms in 80% of patients for 5 years or more. Operative mortality is < 2% but this increases to 3–5% for repeat operations and to 10% in those over 80 years of age. Perioperative myocardial infarction occurs in 4–5% of cases.

Compared with PCI, surgery leads to a more complete revascularization and to a reduced intervention rate. PCI is a less traumatic procedure with a shorter hospital stay and a more rapid return to normal activities. PCI and CABG are, however, complementary. PCI may delay or prevent the need for CABG and may deal with recurrent problems after CABG.

Morbidity

The aftercare is helped by a full and detailed explanation in the preoperative period, reinforced by booklets and videos.

Problems encountered include sternum, back and leg pain, with muscular pain often recurring over 2–3 months (analgesia and anti-inflammatory agents may be necessary). Neurological problems have been reported in 5–6%, with visual disturbances in up to 20%. However, major residual disability affects only 1–2%. Psychiatric morbidity is related to preoperative psychiatric and social maladjustment, neurological personality traits and a previous history of psychiatric illness, and not to the operation itself. Previous peptic ulceration may be exacerbated, and proton pump inhibitors (PPIs) are used for perioperative protection.

After cardiac surgery, a period of 2–3 months to recover and rehabilitate is strongly advised. Return to work is possible in 3 months and driving a motor car at 1 month (though heavy front-wheel drive may give chest wall pain). For holders of heavy goods vehicle or public service vehicle driving licences, a detailed evaluation will be needed after 6 weeks including an exercise ECG (see Table 11).

Table 11   UK guidelines for driving

Cardiovascular disorders	Group 1 ordinary entitlement	Group 2 vocational entitlement
Angina **stable/unstable**	*Driving must cease when symptoms occur at rest or at the wheel* Driving may recommence when satisfactory symptom control is achieved Driver and Vehicle Licensing Agency need not be notified	*Refusal or revocation with continuing symptoms (treated and/or untreated)* Relicensing may be permitted when free from angina for at least 6 weeks provided that the exercise test requirements can be met and there is no other disqualifying condition
Angioplasty/stent	*Driving must cease for at least 1 week* Driving may recommence thereafter provided there is no other disqualifying condition Driver and Vehicle Licensing Agency need not be notified	*Disqualifies from driving for at least 6 weeks* Relicensing may be permitted thereafter provided the exercise test requirements can be met and there is no other disqualifying condition
Myocardial **infarction/CABG**	*Driving must cease for* *at least 4 weeks* Driving may recommence thereafter provided there is no other disqualifying condition Driver and Vehicle Licensing Agency need not be notified	As angioplasty stent

A rehabilitation programme is strongly recommended after CABG, in order to promote confidence and exercise ability, and to afford the opportunity for communication and discussion of problems and objectives. Most patients do well and return to normal activities at 2 months. Sex can be resumed as soon as wished—advice on muscular pain and positions may be needed.

If symptoms return after CABG, they may be controlled by drugs or PCI; however, a referral to the hospital is advised for detailed evaluation.

- Patients must be discharged after surgery with their necessary medical therapy including lipid-lowering drugs and antihypertensives
- General practitioners need to ensure that appropriate therapy remains in place and is regularly monitored

Conduits

Arterial grafts are preferable because of their better long-term patency when compared with vein grafts. It is now routine to use the left internal mammary artery for the left coronary artery.

Graft patency depends initially (in the first 14 days) on thrombosis, and it is determined by technical limitations (e.g. small diseased vessels); in the long term it depends more on lipid-lowering therapy. All patients should be prescribed aspirin or clopidogrel. Figures for vein graft failure of 50% at 10 years have improved with an aggressive lipid-lowering approach. All patients should be on statins. The left internal mammary artery has a 95% patency at 15 years—radial artery 89% at 5 years. Total arterial revascularization may confer long- term benefit but radial artery grafts may stenose in the presence of moderate native coronary stenoses.

Cost

Over 2 years PCI is 80% of the cost of CABG. PCI is more likely to incur early costs due to restenosis and CABG late costs due to vein graft failure. Long-term studies will be influenced by risk-factor modification but both groups will be likely to need further intervention (treatments are palliative not curative).

Specific points

- 5-year survival after CABG is 94%, 10-year survival is 84%
- 10-year survival is 69% in those who continue to smoke
- Abnormal lipids are a major risk for atheroma development and new lesions are reduced to 14% in native vessels and 16% in vein grafts if lipid levels are vigorously reduced by drugs; this compares to 40% and 35%, respectively, when treated by diet alone
- Drugs may be inadvertently stopped at surgery, and review of lipid profiles and hypertensive care is essential

Table 12   Evidence-based management of stable angina

Treatment	Reduces cardiac events (death or myocardial infarction)	Relieves symptoms	Comment
Aspirin	Yes	No	75 mg once daily
Statins	Yes	No	Target is LDL ≤ 2.0 mmol/l
ACE inhibitors	Yes	No	Greatest benefit in high-risk cases
Beta-blockers	Yes (post MI, cardiac failure)	Yes	Use optimally (e.g. atenolol 100 mg once daily)
HRT	No	No	Not recommended for cardiac benefit
Nitrates, potassium activators	No	Yes	Effective for symptom relief
Calcium antagonists: verapamil, diltiazem	Yes	Yes	Alternatives to beta blockers
Other calcium antagonists	No	Yes	Symptom relief
Trimetazidine	Yes (some evidence in cardiac failure)	Yes	Minimal adverse effects. Effective in combination therapy
Ivabradine	No (trial ongoing)	Yes	Alternative to beta-blockade
Ranolazine	No	Yes	US only
PCI	No	Yes	Effective when medicine fails
Stents	No	Yes	As PCI
CABG	Yes	Yes	Selected cases
Antioxidants	No	No	
Stop smoking	Yes	Yes	Cheap therapy

Minimally invasive surgery

The use of 'off-pump' coronary surgery was developed to reduce perioperative morbidity, especially cognitive impairment. The proposed advantages included less pain, less bleeding, a shorter hospital stay and, by avoiding bypass, less chance of neurological problems and lower cost. At the present time, trials have identified no difference between off- and on-pump CABG at 30 days regarding mortality, MI, stroke or renal dysfunction, but hospital stay and rate of atrial fibrillation was less off-pump. Effects on cognitive function have been inconclusive and there is therefore no evidence base for off-pump use to prevent cognitive decline.

Key points

- CABG relieves symptoms when angina is refractory to medical treatment
- CABG may improve prognosis, depending on the anatomy
- CABG is an option when PCI is unsuccessful or not possible
- Long-term survival depends on control of risk factors (especially lipid levels)

Stable angina—the choices summarized

- The objective is to relieve symptoms and lengthen life by practising evidence-based medicine (Table 12)
- A good history is supplemented by stress testing to identify those at greatest risk
- General measures are important—stopping smoking, using aspirin, controlling lipids and blood pressure, avoiding obesity and increasing physical exercise
- CABG is recommended for those at high risk for prognostic as well as symptomatic reasons
- Medical treatment and PCI are effective means of relieving symptoms, with PCI having a principal role when medical therapy is ineffective
- PCI may be an alternative to CABG when operative risks are considered too high because of other medical problems (e.g. severe lung disease)
- The treatments are complementary and not mutually exclusive (e.g. a stenotic vein graft can be corrected by PCI)
- The general practitioner, by having in mind the two objectives of improving prognosis and relieving symptoms, can advise the patient appropriately and refer the patient for further advice when needed

Refractory angina

When angina markedly limits ordinary physical activity or occurs on minimal activity or at rest, in spite of optimal medical therapy, it is by definition refractory. Since both PCI and CABG are effective in relieving symptoms, these options should have been excluded by experienced interventional cardiologists or cardiac surgeons, with their decision based on a recent coronary angiogram. In one study of transmyocardial laser revascularization, 71 of 117 patients (62%), who were initially referred because of refractory angina, responded to either a change in their medication, PCI or CABG.

Establishing that angina is truly refractory to conventional therapy requires a detailed evaluation of each individual patient.

Any pain felt must be a direct result of ischaemia. Musculoskeletal pains and gastric symptoms (e.g. pain from a hiatus hernia) are common and need to be excluded. Any precipitating causes should be excluded. If hypertension is present, has it been effectively controlled to a target of 130/80 mmHg or less? Have the preferred agents for angina and hypertension (beta-blockers and calcium antagonists) been optimally utilized? A check should be made for anaemia, aortic valve disease, rapid or slow arrhythmias (especially atrial fibrillation in the elderly) and thyrotoxicosis.

The patient needs to take medication and to take it correctly. Sometimes complex regimens may be too demanding. Depression caused by their condition may lead to poor adherence on the part of patients to therapy. Also, the medication has to be the optimal dosage. Conventional agents (beta-blockers, nitrates, calcium antagonists, Ivabradine and potassium-channel activators) act haemodynamically. Once the maximum haemodynamic effect has been achieved, the addition of further similarly acting agents presents no advantage. Optimal dose haemodynamic monotherapy occasionally benefits from the addition of a second agent (e.g. beta-blocker plus nitrate) but triple or quadruple therapy confers no additional benefit and may actually increase symptoms. Metabolic therapy with trimetazidine may be effective when added to conventional haemodynamic agents.

To get the full benefit of any conventional therapy, cigarette smoking should stop, advice should be given about obesity and activity should be encouraged. If the patients are anxious or depressed, appropriate counselling should be organized. Lipid-lowering therapy should be optimally deployed to maximize the benefits of slowing disease progression or inducing regression, which may lead to long-term symptomatic benefit.

A comprehensive rehabilitation programme including education, close supervision of lifestyle advice and cognitive behaviour therapy may be helpful and should be explored.

Spinal cord stimulation may have a positive effect on symptoms with few adverse effects. Small numbers have been evaluated and a placebo effect cannot be discounted though experienced centres report increased treadmill exercise time. Overall it is unproven.

Enhanced external counterpulsation (EECP) uses compressed air applied via cuffs to the legs timed to synchronize with diastole to propel blood back to the coronary arteries. At the end of diastole the cuffs are deflated, reducing vascular impedence.

The technique is well tolerated (35 hours over about 6 weeks) but reported decreases in symptoms and increased exercise time to ischaemia do not appear to be significantly different from placebo.

Transmyocardial revascularization provides no advantage over a surgical sham procedure. Gene therapy leading to angiogenesis and agents to improve endothelial function are also being evaluated.

In summary, refractory angina must be carefully defined. Optimal use of all treatment modalities needs to be rigorously applied. While new techniques are being developed, already established therapies must not be neglected—when fully utilized, clinical benefit may follow.

Coronary disease in women

CAD is the commonest cause of death for women. Approximately seven times as many women die of CAD as die of breast cancer. Though less frequent under the age of 65 years, it is a diagnosis that should always be considered in the presence of chest pain. Women with CAD present with angina more frequently than with myocardial infarction, but their pain is often atypical and difficult to pin down. Exercise tests are more often false positive for CAD than in men, especially in young women, who have a low incidence of CAD. Over the age of 65 years, exercise tests are more accurate, reflecting the increased incidence of CAD in the older female population (about 1 in 3).

Women with CAD are more frequently diabetic and/or hypertensive than other women. Cigarette smoking is an important risk factor, which is increasing in young women as a result of 'clever' targeted advertising against a background of increasing social pressure. Hyperlipidaemia should be looked for; however, the full lipid profile must always be measured since women have a higher HDL until the age of 65 years, and lowering this will be counterproductive. The low-dose contraceptive pills do not appear to increase the incidence of CAD, though smoking while on the pill is a cause for concern and should always be counselled against. Women benefit from treatment the same as men, but they are often older at presentation and have more severe disease; this, combined with naturally smaller coronary arteries, may contribute to the slightly higher complication and mortality rate noted for PCI and CABG in women.

- HRT is not indicated for the prevention of CAD

Women do not always receive the same treatment as men for a given cardiac problem. The question of a sex bias is disputed but is almost certainly real, though there is always the possibility of age bias (women are older at presentation).

- Bias in management invariably is linked to resources available
- This may lead to ageism
- As a consequence (women live longer), there will appear to be sexism
- However a more conservative approach in women may be to their advantage rather than disadvantage (see COURAGE trial, page 20)

Coronary disease in the elderly

The elderly may have different priorities and be more concerned about being a burden on others. They are more willing to accept mild to moderate angina on medical therapy rather than to consider an interventional route.

The elderly have more diffuse disease affecting all three major coronary arteries. Left ventricular function is often depressed. Co-morbid conditions may limit their mobility (e.g. arthritis, which in turn will limit their exercise ability in daily life and so their capability of performing an exercise ECG).

'Young for their age' patients above 70 years should be offered the same therapeutic options as younger patients because they benefit just as much, although complications after CABG are more frequent.

With age, drug bioavailability changes, and dose modification is often necessary because sensitivity increases. Always commence with low doses in the elderly, titrating cautiously to effect. Because of polypharmacy in this age group, adherence to medication is variable, so it is important to advise on the importance of not stopping drugs abruptly without medical advice.

Always be on the lookout for other causes of angina, especially poorly controlled atrial fibrillation and aortic valve disease.

The elderly are more sensitive to haemodynamic side effects of beta-blockers and metabolic agents such as trimetazidine may be better tolerated.

Specific areas

Unstable angina

Variant angina

Chest pain with normal
coronary arteries

Referring patients

Practical points

Unstable angina

Unstable angina is a new presentation or the development of angina that represents a volatile midpoint between stable angina and myocardial infarction. The key characteristics are:

- new angina (<1 month) at a low workload (22.5–45 metres walking on the flat)
- worsening of stable angina for no obvious reason
- angina at rest

Diagnosis

Out of hospital, patients can be divided into low-, medium- and high-risk categories using the criteria laid out in Table 13. In addition, screening for elevation of troponin T or I identifies high-risk cases. This may be possible out of hospital using rapid desktop analysis.

Management

To optimize management, medium- and high-risk cases need hospital care and should be admitted as soon as the diagnosis has been made, whereas low-risk cases can be evaluated initially and treated by the general practitioner. Before admission to hospital, medium- and high-risk patients should be prescribed the following:

- aspirin 300 mg, crunched and swallowed plus clopidogrel 300–600 mg loading dose
- glyceryl trinitrate
- opiates if the pain is severe (plus an antiemetic)
- intravenous furosemide (20–40 mg) if there is pulmonary oedema

Low-risk patients can be managed out of hospital (Figure 15). However, if a rapid access chest pain clinic is available, an immediate referral is recommended and the patient will usually be seen within 48 hours. Management should be started by checking for precipitating causes, such as anaemia, hypertension, or tachyarrhythmias (especially atrial fibrillation in the elderly). Unless contraindicated, an initial dose of aspirin 300 mg followed by 75 mg per day should be initiated and sublingual nitrates should be prescribed.

Table 13 Unstable angina: independent criteria for patient categorization

Low-risk cases
- New-onset or worsening exertional angina
- Increasing angina frequency, severity or duration
- No episodes of prolonged pain (over 20 minutes) or pain at rest
- No ECG changes from previous recordings or a normal ECG

Medium-risk cases
- Rest angina in the last 2 weeks but now settled or responding to glyceryl trinitrate
- Nocturnal angina
- New onset of severe angina in the past 2 weeks at a low workload (<22.5 metres walking on the flat)
- ECG evidence of ischaemia not previously known
- Age over 65 years

High-risk cases
- Chest pain of over 20 minutes' duration
- Pain after recent infarction
- Evidence of pulmonary oedema
- Angina with new or worsening mitral regurgitation
- Hypotension
- New ischaemic (ST segment) changes on the ECG

If suitable, beta-blockade should be started (e.g. atenolol 50–100 mg per day). If beta-blockers are contraindicated, a heart-rate-lowering calcium antagonist such as diltiazem should be used.

All calcium antagonists have a therapeutic role in stable angina, either as monotherapy or in combination. However, dihydropyridines have a more pronounced peripheral vasodilating effect and can cause a reflex tachycardia that is potentially threatening in unstable angina: this risk can be avoided by co-prescribing with beta-blockers.

Although long-acting dihydropyridines such as amlodipine are less likely to induce a tachycardia because of their slow onset of action, it is still wise to avoid any risk by co-prescribing beta-blockers.

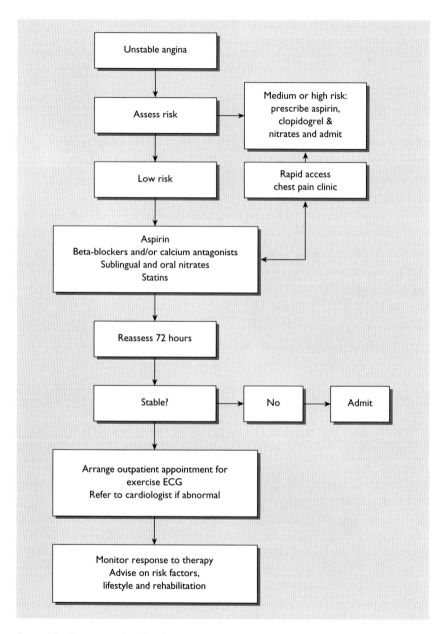

Figure 15 Treatment algorithm for unstable angina out-of-hospital assessment.

Isosorbide mononitrate can be used alone when there is known left ventricular dysfunction, but it should also be considered as combination therapy in all patients on beta-blockers or calcium antagonists because of its additive benefit.

Follow-up

Patients should be reassessed after 48–72 hours and admitted to hospital if not stable. Any new changes in the ECG should be noted and the patient advised to go to the emergency medical department of a local hospital if symptoms worsen in the mean time.

If the patient stabilizes, medical therapy should be continued, adjusting the dose according to the degree of effect.

An outpatient assessment for an exercise ECG is necessary to establish risk status and the need for angiography with a view to PCI or CABG.

It is important to educate patients on the necessity of seeking help if the symptoms change in the future or if they fail to respond rapidly to sublingual nitrates.

Unstable angina will either settle over 4–6 weeks and become stable angina or else threaten to progress to non-fatal or fatal myocardial infarction.

An initial medical approach followed by risk stratification and selective intervention or intervention if symptoms persist inspite of optimal medical therapy.

Key points

- Unstable angina patients may be at increased risk of myocardial infarction and death
- Antiplatelet and anti-ischaemic agents are the mainstays of out-of-hospital therapy
- Most patients settle with conservative regimens
- Risk stratification is essential
- High-risk cases benefit from PCI or CABG
- If in doubt admit as an emergency
- Use rapid access chest pain clinics where available

Variant angina

The term 'variant angina' refers to patients who get pain at rest with ST elevation on the ECG. It may occur at the same time of day (the most common being night and

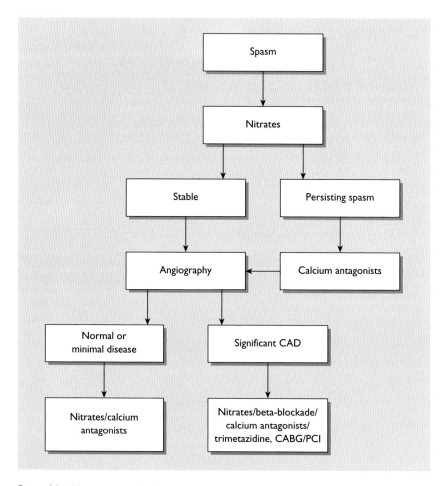

Figure 16   *Management plan for variant angina.*

early morning) and be associated with syncope. Exertional angina may or may not coexist.

The cause is coronary artery spasm. There was a 9% death rate and a 38% infarct rate at 2 years in Prinzmetal's original series. If the coronary anatomy is normal, cardiac events occur in 8% of patients; if CAD exists, cardiac events occur in 30%.

These (old) figures may be influenced by newer drugs and techniques.

Management

A management strategy is shown in Figure 16. Referral is recommended.

Note that nitrates and calcium antagonists are first-choice agents. The condition should be managed initially as unstable angina. Existing beta-blockade should be continued, especially if CAD is known to exist; it should be avoided otherwise (the unopposed alpha-effects may lead to vasoconstriction). Aspirin should be used as for unstable angina. Trimetazidine can be used as it has no vaso-constrictive properties.

When the angina is stable, proceed to angiography. If significant CAD exists, beta blockade may be added at this point.

CABG has a higher risk here than for stable angina, and spasm may recur post-operatively. Continue antispasm drugs postoperatively (e.g. diltiazem plus mononitrates).

Chest pain with normal coronary arteries

It is an understatement to say this is a difficult group to manage. Syndrome X is the association of angina chest pain with angiographically normal coronary arteries and an abnormal exercise ECG. In patients with non-cardiac or atypical pain it is important to rule out oesophageal disease. Hyperventilation and psychological disorders are also common.

In cases where ischaemia can be induced, the possibility of endothelial dysfunction arises. As the incidence of syndrome X is greater in women and invariably presents after the menopause, oestrogen deficiency, which is known to cause endothelial dysfunction, has been suggested as a possible cause. There is evidence that HRT may be beneficial.

Patients can be reassured about the good prognosis, since the mortality and infarct rate is <1% over 10 years. Unfortunately pain continues to restrict 75% of patients, with 50% being unemployed or disabled. These patients are a particular problem for the general practitioner, since treatment is difficult and invariably 'hit and miss' and no specific hospital therapy is available.

- Always reassure the patient
  Rule out an oesophageal cause—try a course of a proton pump inhibitor (e.g. omeprazole)
- Try HRT if there are no contraindications
- Typical pain may respond to conventional antianginal therapy
- 'Ring the changes' but try to avoid more than two drugs at a time—'switch therapy'
- Smoking should be strongly discouraged
- Be frank with the patient—let him or her know it is a difficult problem but emphasize it is not life threatening
- One of my patients improved after years of disability when I tried adding in sildenafil—not an evidence-based therapy, but this is not an evidence-based condition

Referring patients

In general, refer:

- when not sure of the diagnosis
- to exclude other causes (e.g. aortic valve disease)
- if unstable and not low risk
- if symptomatic on optimal medical treatment
- to identify those at prognostic risk (e.g. by exercise ECG)
- for guidance on overall management if unsure of the options

Practical points

Stable angina

- Treating angina is a team approach between the patient, the doctor and nurse
- Symptoms can be controlled with nitrates, nicorandil, beta-blockers, ivabradine, calcium antagonists, trimetazidine and ranolazine
- Most nitrates are subject to hepatic metabolism but this can be avoided by using a mononitrate preparation
- Beta-blockade needs to be used to optimal doses and not reduced when asymptomatic resting bradycardia occurs
- When beta-blockers are contraindicated or not tolerated, use calcium antagonists or ivabradine and/or nitrates and/or trimetazidine
- Peripheral side effects of beta-blockers can be reduced by dose reduction, using an agent with PAA or changing to calcium antagonists or ivabradine
- Diltiazem, verapamil and amlodipine are effective as monotherapy. Nifedipine and amlodipine, by avoiding conduction interaction, are safer and effective in combination with beta-blockade, whereas diltiazem can be used cautiously in combination (verapamil is not recommended)
- Most adverse effects are caused by inappropriate patient selection; do not take chances
- Metabolic agents (e.g. trimetazidine) are effective in relieving symptoms as monotherapy or in combination
- Ivabradine is a therapeutic alternative to beta-blockers
- PCI is successful in 95% of patients, but restenosis remains a problem in spite of DES
- PCI may be effective when medical therapy for moderate or severe angina is unsuccessful
- Stents reduce restenosis after PCI from 30% to 10% and are more effective for vein graft lesions. Their use is widespread
- Surgery is more effective than PCI in relieving symptoms, with less reintervention long term
- Surgery not only prolongs life for some patients but also relieves symptoms in over 80% of those who fail to respond to medicine
- Age should be no barrier to surgery or PCI if the patient is otherwise well
- Surgical mortality averages <2%. For the family, however, a death is 100%
- Aspirin (75 mg once daily) is advised for all suitable cases
- Lipid-lowering therapy is advised for all cases

Unstable angina

- Unstable angina is effort pain of recent onset, a changing pattern of angina or angina at rest
- Hospital admission is advised for medium- and high-risk cases
- Low-risk cases need risk stratification out of hospital (but if unsure admit)

Variant angina

- Coronary artery spasm may occur with and without CAD
- It is the cause of variant angina
- It is involved in 30–40% of cases of unstable angina
- The most rapidly effective drugs are the intravenous nitrates
- Calcium antagonists are frequently helpful, either alone or in combination with nitrates and/or trimetazidine
- Angiography is advised to rule out significant coronary disease
- If surgery is performed, spasm may still recur, so nitrates and calcium antagonists may be used postoperatively, even if the patient is apparently free of pain

Often overlooked

- CAD occurs in premenopausal women also
- Lipids need monitoring
- The effect on the family—the need for rehabilitation and support
- The effect on the children of parents with heart disease

Further reading

Fox K, Garcia MA, Ardissino D, et al; Task Force on the Management of Stable Angina Pectoris of the European Society of Cardiology; ESC Committee for Practice Guidelines (CPG). Guidelines on the management of stable angina pectoris, executive summary: the Task Force on the Management of Stable Angina Pectoris of the European Society of Cardiology. Eur Heart J 2006; 27: 1341–81.

SIGN 96: Management of stable angina. 2007: www.sign.ac.uk.

Wenger NK, Collins P (eds). Women and Heart Disease. London: Taylor and Francis, 2005.

Index

N.B. Page numbers in *italic* denote figures or tables.

morbidity 68, 70
vs CABG 66
vs drug therapy 66
see also balloon angioplasty
pericarditis *16*
phosphodiesterase type 5 (PDE5)
  inhibitors 43–4, *44*
physical activity 37, 38, 73
  after surgery 70
pindolol *51*
plain old balloon angioplasty
  (POBA) 63, *64*
POBA (plain old balloon angioplasty)
  see balloon angioplasty
positron emission tomography
  (PET) 26–7
postprandial angina 14
potassium channel activators 59, *71*, 73
pravastatin *42*
pre-infarction angina *see* unstable angina
prevalence 4, 22
prevention 36–42
Prinzmetal's angina
  see variant angina
prognosis 1
  improvement of 20
propranolol *51*, 52, 54
psychological morbidity after surgery 68
pulmonary hypertension 17
pulmonary oedema 78
pulmonary pain *16*

quality of life 4

ranolazine 60, *71*, 86
referral 85
  guidelines 33
refractory angina 73–4
restenosis 67
revascularization
  laser 73
  recommendation 21
rosuvastatin *42*
rotational devices 67–8

screening 31–2
second wind angina 15
sestamibi imaging 26
sex differences
  see gender differences
sexual activity 43–4, *44*
  drug-induced effects 43
sildenafil (Viagra) 43–4, *44*, 84
silent myocardial ischaemia 25, 33
simvastatin *42*
single photon emission
  computed tomography
  (SPECT) 25, 26
smoking 36
  cessation *71*, 73
  and chest pain 84
  women *37*
spinal cord stimulation 74
ST segment modification 23–4
stable angina
  aetiology 18
  angina of effort *8*
  auscultation 17–18
  definition 7, 9
  driving after *69*
  examination 18
    checklist *18*
  management
    choices 72
    evidence-based *71*
  practical points 86
statins 20
  beneficial actions 40, 42
  evidence of benefits 40–2
  guideline targets 41–2
  in stable angina *71*
stenosis 28
stents/stenting 63, 66–7, 86
  driving after *69*
  in stable angina *71*
  technique *65*
sternum pain, postoperative 68
stress 38
strokes *39*